Praise for *Meridian Qigong Exercises*

More than twenty years ago, I stepped into my first taiji class with Dr. Yang, in a studio room behind an auto dealership in Andover, Massachusetts. The class began with taiji qigong movements as a way of orienting the students to qi and helping us feel our own body's qi. For me, this was the first time I had ever experienced qi, and thus began my lifelong journey into qigong and taiji. Since that time, Dr. Yang has led the Western community in the exploration of qigong. He has published countless books on the subject, educated by his teaching experience and many translations of ancient documents.

As qigong and "complementary" medicine have grown in popularity in the United States and Europe, Dr. Yang has provided rational, simple explanations for the benefits of qigong movements, breathing, and the mind-body connection. He has explored, taught, and written about countless qigong sets and practices from the medical, martial, and spiritual schools. His clear-eyed insights have opened up this mystical, complex art and mapped many of its secrets to Western science and understanding.

The term *yoga* has evolved in our contemporary culture to describe a wide range of practices and styles—the best of which involve stretching the body while cultivating a mind-body connection. In his latest book, *Meridian Qigong Exercises*, Dr. Yang elucidates a series of simple, accessible stretches that open and activate the body's qi channels and massage the organs. He provides a terrific overview of the health benefits of several of the acupuncture points along the channels. Adding self-massage allows the practitioner to explore these points and their effects.

It has been a great joy for me to study from and develop a friendship with Dr. Yang. The inspiring arc of his career has spanned from his small New England base to a worldwide network of schools and many publications, to his current focus at the YMAA Retreat Center, where he teaches a small group of committed students who spend their days developing the martial, health, and spiritual sides of qigong, taiji, and Shaolin gongfu. All of us are fortunate to have Dr. Yang's formidable intelligence and skills focused on revealing and exploring these great arts. *Meridian Qigong Exercises* is another gift from Dr. Yang in his journey to bring the health benefits of qigong to the Western audience.

Bill Buckley
Registered yoga teacher; certified taijiquan, chin na, and qigong instructor (YMAA); owner and chief instructor at GateWay Taiji, Qigong, and Yoga in Portsmouth, New Hampshire

Early in my training I found my way to the Tai Chi Farm Festival held by the late Master Jou, Tsung Hwa at his farm in Warwick, New Jersey. It was a mecca for those seeking to share their tai chi and qigong experience. Well-known teachers from all over the world gathered to present their teachings as an offering of respect to their beloved friend and colleague, Master Jou. This welcoming environment is where I met Dr. Yang, Jwing-Ming in 1997.

Having studied with several teachers already by that point, Dr. Yang provided a key missing step on my journey. Many teachers at that time were still in the mode of restricting the information they would give out, as if the knowledge were a treasure that shouldn't easily be spent. Dr. Yang was of the opposite mind. If there was a question, he would answer it, and he would answer it completely, all the way to its root, to the place where his mind had taken it on his own inquiry.

It was a stunning revelation to me at the time that a person could and should learn to analyze qigong and decipher its meaning and purpose. That by learning the principles of energy flow and body mechanics, one could determine how a qigong exercise would influence the body. I was hooked. I knew that if I spent the time to learn the principles that Dr. Yang taught, I would have the "road map," as he calls it, to find my way. I have been his student ever since and received master-level certification in qigong through his school, YMAA, in 2012. Dr. Yang's open style of deep inquiry and sharing has inspired me to continually raise the bar of what I learn and teach, pushing me to be a better student and teacher as the years go on.

Dr. Yang has a very rare interest and talent for translating ancient Chinese documents to bring their knowledge to the modern world. The singularity of this talent is not just in the translation process but also in his ability to interpret the deeper meaning of the words. This requires the unique ability, gleaned from his many years of study, to experiment with the material to plumb its depths and fully bring it to life.

Dr. Yang has gone one giant step further over his long career. He has added to the ancient wisdom by creating his own styles that are based on his training and experience and profound understanding in order to fill in the gaps of what modern qigong has to offer.

Dr. Yang's experience makes him eminently qualified to create a new style of qigong: Twelve Meridian Ground Qigong Yoga. This new qigong integrates the methods of increasing circulation through the muscles and joints interpreted from his experience with muscle/tendon changing qigong (see Dr. Yang's *Qigong, The Secret of Youth: Da Mo's Muscle/Tendon Changing and Marrow/Brain Washing Classics,* 2000) and the methods of self-massage utilizing acupressure points (see his *Qigong Massage,* 2005).

Our lifestyles create challenges the ancients never had. In my more than twenty years of experience teaching qigong and tai chi and practicing qi healing, I have learned many qigong styles and healers' techniques. The tools in this book unveil a new powerfully relaxing and accessible healing form that fills a missing niche, the transition from being asleep at night into our daily activities and then again, from that busy day into a restful state in order to promote healing sleep at night.

Having practiced and taught Dr. Yang's joint movements and self-massage techniques for more than eighteen years, I know that his methods are very effective and healing for the body. Having his techniques finally available in one accessible flowing routine that can be done in bed makes it so easy to add healing and self-care to our lives. The techniques in this book are a perfect addition to anyone's personal practice to improve health, reduce stress, and relieve pain.

Once again, I am inspired by Dr. Yang's continuing efforts to push the boundaries of qigong and make it available to us all.

Lisa B. O'Shea
Certified qigong master
Rochester, New York

Meridian Qigong Exercises

COMBINING QIGONG, YOGA, AND ACUPRESSURE

DR. YANG, JWING-MING

YMAA Publication Center
Wolfeboro, NH USA

YMAA Publication Center, Inc.
PO Box 480
Wolfeboro, New Hampshire, 03894
1-800-669-8892 • info@ymaa.com • www.ymaa.com

ISBN: 9781594394133 (print) • ISBN: 9781594394140 (ebook)

Edited by David Silver
Copy edit and caption edit by Leslie Takao
Cover design by Axie Breen
Photographs by Nathan Rosen unless otherwise noted
This book typeset in 12 pt. Adobe Garamond
Typesetting by Westchester Publishing Services
Anatomy drawings adapted from Shutterstock.com

20191208

Publisher's Cataloging in Publication

Names: Yang, Jwing-Ming, 1946- author.
Title: Meridian qigong exercises : combining qigong, yoga, and acupressure / by Dr. Yang, Jwing-Ming.
Description: Wolfeboro, NH USA : YMAA Publication Center, [2016] | "A simple lying-down routine for
    everyone"—Cover. | Includes bibliographical references.
Identifiers: ISBN: 9781594394133 (print) | 978159439140 (ebook) | LCCN: 2016962075
Subjects: LCSH: Qi gong. | Stretching exercises. | Yoga. | Acupressure. | Qi (Chinese philosphy) |
    Mind and body. | Medicine, Chinese. | Holistic medicine. | BISAC: HEALTH & FITNESS / Exercise. |
    HEALTH & FITNESS / Healing. | HEALTH & FITNESS / Yoga. | SPORTS & RECREATION /
    Martial Arts & Self-Defense.
Classification: LCC: RA781.8 .Y3635 2016 | DDC: 613.7/148— dc23

Dedications

To my three masters:
Cheng, Gin-Gsao (曾金灶)—White Crane (白鶴拳)
Li, Mao-Ching (李茂清)—Long Fist (長拳)
Kao, Tao (高濤)—Taijiquan (太極拳)

My wife, Mei-Ling (美玲)

and

My three children, James (志堅), Kathy (愷怡), and Nicholas (志豪)

and

All students and friends I have had in the last forty years who always
gave me inspiration and encouragement

Table of Contents

Foreword

This book is special.

Dr. Yang's previous work has presented detailed instruction and theory for all of the most popular qigong forms, tracing back the roots of the art in the process. He has clarified, simplified, and preserved these classics forever, poring over all available documents in order to make his teaching as accurate and effective as possible.

He has given the world expositions on the two-thousand-year-old Daoist "Five Animal Sports"; Bodhidharma's Buddhist "Muscle/Tendon Changing" and "Brain/Marrow Washing Qigong" from 550 CE; and the popular thousand-year-old series known as the "Eight Brocades." He has passed down the ancient Shaolin White Crane qigong system from his own personal lineage that he mastered in his youth during thirteen years of ongoing study with his Master Cheng, Gin-Gsao (曾金灶). He has transmitted the most comprehensive qi theory as it pertains to taijiquan and all martial arts, after decades of research and practice. One of Dr. Yang's major accomplishments has been compiling, translating, and cross-referencing hundreds of documents in his ongoing creation of a unified theory of qigong.

Now nearing the age of seventy, Dr. Yang gives us *Meridian Qigong Exercises*, the book and companion video, his own personal daily qigong regimen, combining the most effective movements from multiple disciplines. This routine can be done on a chair or in bed, and it systematically improves the function of your entire physical and energetic body. I highly recommend this instant classic.

David Silver
Cape Cod Qigong
Cape Cod, Massachusetts

Foreword

In traditional Chinese medicine, the most important key to attaining health and healing is the free flow of qi in the body's meridian system. Much like a river that needs to flow from a mountaintop to the ocean and cycle back again through evaporation and condensation, qi needs to flow smoothly and abundantly through a continuous cycle in our bodies. This cycle promotes the cleansing, detoxification, and nourishing of our internal organs and is crucial for maintaining good health. When the organ system becomes imbalanced, toxins can accumulate and block the qi flow. This blockage is what leads to various ailments, pains, and discomforts in our bodies.

Meridian qigong can play a major role in regulating our qi in accordance with the body's natural rhythm. Simple exercises, such as wiggling your toes from the moment you wake up to pressing acupressure points on your hands and feet before you sleep, can help change the way you feel during the day and at night. These exercises can be easily integrated into your daily routines, such as while brushing your teeth or taking a shower. Over time, this practice builds awareness of the body's meridians and how they relate to different signs and symptoms. With regular practice, you will naturally learn to recognize these connections and know how to remove irregularities in your own body's energy.

I was first introduced to qigong by my father when I was eleven years old. Since then, the more I learned about qigong, the more I discovered how it could help me develop a stronger body, mind, and spirit. Also, the healing effects of qigong fascinated me. This interest eventually led me to pursue my degrees in clinical exercise physiology and traditional Chinese medicine. My studies gave me a systematic way to better understand the intricacies of qi, specifically how qi imbalances can lead to various illnesses. With this deeper understanding of how qi works in our bodies and in nature, I developed a strong belief that we can and should be very active in our own healing process.

Throughout the years, it has been a great joy of mine to observe the deep and significant impact my father has had on people's lives all over the world. I have been moved by the stories people share with me of how he has helped them better manage their conditions, such as chronic back pain, knee problems, arthritis, asthma, and even cancer. He has made this ancient knowledge of qigong accessible to our modern-day lives. Never has he ceased to amaze me with his innovativeness, pursuit of knowledge, and sincerity to share. He has been, and remains to be, the source of my inspiration.

I invite you to discover the ways in which qigong has inspired and impacted my life, and I hope it can do the same for yours.

Kathy Yang
MSc in Chinese medicine and BSc in traditional Chinese medicine
from Middlesex University, London, UK

Bachelor of medicine from Beijing University of Chinese Medicine, Beijing, China
BSc in clinical exercise physiology from Boston University, Boston, Massachusetts, USA

Preface

Over the last fifty years, I have been searching for and compiling information on the qigong and yoga (which is essentially Indian qigong) that can be effectively used to benefit today's society. Our lifestyle today is very different from that of a hundred years ago. We are all busy and have less time. In addition, due to pollution in our air, water, and even the energy itself, this world has become the most difficult, contaminated, and harmful living environment ever existing in human history. In this situation, the body is constantly detoxing, and people commonly develop abnormal qi (energy) circulation patterns. For this reason, qigong and yoga practice have become more important than ever. Because of its emphasis on maintaining smooth qi and blood circulation, these internal arts have been commonly used to maintain body health and extend life span. With regular practice, a practitioner will be able to regulate the abnormal qi circulation and strengthen the body's vital force.

These qigong exercises focus on opening the twelve primary qi channels (meridians) in the early morning right after you wake up. When you sleep, your body's hormones are produced, and part of their function is to expedite the body's metabolism. But when we metabolize unclean food, water, and air, the body begins to accumulate toxic material. Early morning exercises and drinking water immediately after waking up are the crucial keys to help remove the toxins built up during sleep.

In this book, I have compiled these qigong movements from my more than fifty years of practicing and teaching experience. These qigong exercises focus on cleansing the body's twelve qi channels so the irregular qi circulation can be corrected. Practicing daily will help you regain your health and maintain your vital energy.

In addition, I also introduce some effective and easy self-massage routines, using tui na and cavity acupressure techniques that allow you to enhance the qi circulation in the channels. These cavities are selected from traditional Chinese medicine and commonly used in acupuncture.

Once you have practiced for a while with this book and companion DVD, you will be able to comprehend the theory behind it and may even create new movements that are more suitable for your lifestyle, body shape, and environment. These exercises only offer you some ideas and references to get started. You should keep your mind open and dare to experiment with new exercises, while listening to your body's subtle feedback. I sincerely hope that *Meridian Qigong Exercises* is able to inspire you and make your life healthier.

Dr. Yang, Jwing-Ming
YMAA California Retreat Center
September 15, 2013

Chapter 1: Meridian Qigong Exercises

1-1. Introduction

Before you begin practicing, there are a few points you should understand. These exercises are designed to be done in bed, and ideally, you'll be able to memorize them so you can practice without the book or DVD. But at first, you'll need the book or the video by your side. Before we start exercising, let me explain the benefits and the best time to practice.

Benefits of Exercises

To gain the most benefits from the meridian qigong exercises and acupressure, it is highly recommended that you practice all of the movements. These movements are designed in an order ideal to motivate the qi and blood circulation. However, if you feel the number of repetitions is too many or too few, you may adjust to fit what you need.

Benefits

1. Increasing Health and Longevity

The benefits you can gain from these exercises are not only to maintain your general health but also to slow down your aging process. The key of reaching these goals is to keep practicing regularly so that the body is able to get rid of the waste, and you can regain your vital force.

2. Relaxing and Reconditioning Your Torso (Spine and Lower Back)

Many exercises focus on torso movements that can not only loosen up the torso but also rebuild its strength. In Chinese medicine, the muscles/tendons that wrap around the torso are considered an organ called triple burner (sanjiao, 三焦). When these wrapping muscles/tendons are loosened, the internal organs can be relaxed. Consequently, the qi and blood can smoothly circulate in the organs. In addition, through these exercises, you will also condition your torso and spine, especially the lower back. Therefore, to those who already have spine or lower back problems, these exercises will help you to regain health.

3. Opening the Twelve Primary Qi Channels (Meridians)

All exercises are designed to open up or to reactivate the qi's circulation in the twelve primary qi channels. Once these channels are wide opened, the qi can circulate abundantly and smoothly. This will thus enhance the blood circulation as well. Qi and blood circulation is the crucial key to getting rid of the body's toxins, especially when done in the early morning, right after waking up. In addition, if you practice before your sleep, you will loosen up the body and improve the qi and blood circulation. This will help you get rid of the toxins that have accumulated from daytime physical activities. Practicing before you sleep will provide a good circulating condition for the body's metabolism during your sleep. However, you may experience that it is harder to fall asleep because the enhanced circulation may excite your mind and body.

4. Strengthening Internal Organs

Another benefit of enhancing qi circulation in the twelve primary qi channels is to recondition your internal organs such as the kidneys, spleen, liver, lungs, and heart. When the qi's circulation in the twelve primary qi channels is enhanced due to the more abundant qi circulation provided, the internal organs can be conditioned and rebuilt. It is known in Chinese qigong practice that the crucial key of rebuilding the internal organs' healthy condition is through abundant qi circulation. After all, if there is not enough energy circulating in the internal organs, then there is nothing that can be used to recondition the organs.

5. Improving Joint Problems

Many exercises focus on stretching and exercising the joints. When you lie down, the physical body is relaxed, especially the joints. Therefore, it is the best position for stretching and exercising the joints and enhancing the qi's circulation in the joints. This is the crucial key to healing and reconditioning.

6. Improving the Digestive System

Some of the exercises emphasize the abdominal area's movement and massage. Through these exercises and massage, the qi will circulate following the bowel system. This is the key to improving the function of the digestive system.

7. Preventing Prostate and Breast Cancers

Through the shoulder and hip joint exercises, the qi stagnant around the breast and prostate areas can be removed. In Chinese medicine, it is recognized that smooth qi circulation is the key to preventing or treating cancers. Naturally, correct exercises and massage are the two most common treatments for cancer problems.

I hope this introduction has convinced you of the effectiveness and the benefits of meridian qigong. Please allow at least three months of practice to verify these benefits.

The keys to making this happen are patience and consistence. If you find this is beneficial to you, please introduce these exercises to others such as your friends and family.

Important Points

1. Time of Practice (練習時間)

To gain the most benefit from these exercises, there are three optimal times that you can practice.
A. Right after waking up (剛睡醒)—Best time
B. Right before sleep (睡前)—Second-best time
C. Dusk (傍晚)—Third-best time

2. Do Not Practice with Full or Empty Stomach (不要飽食、空肚)

There are a lot of swaying and circling motions in these exercises. If you have a full stomach when you do these exercises, you will feel very uncomfortable. It is important to feel comfortable and relaxed. Naturally, if you are too hungry, that will also affect your exercises; you should eat a little bit of food first. However, if you feel comfortable right after you wake up, that would be the best time.

3. Drink Plenty of Water (喝水足量)

If you feel thirsty during practice, the waste in your body will not move adequately. Water is a necessary element to help cleanse the body. If you can, place a glass of water next to your bed so you will have it right when you are waking up.

4. Breathe Naturally (呼吸自然)

Breathing is a crucial key to repelling waste in the body. Plenty of oxygen will offer you a high level of metabolism. Therefore, when you practice, you should breathe naturally and deeply. Holding the breath can only cause tightness of the body.

5. Adequate Number of Repetitions (運動量適度)

The right amount of exercise is always the key to progress. Too much will harm you, and too little will not be effective. In addition, you must consider how much time you have. If you rush through, even though you have done a lot of exercises, the result will not be as great as when you take time and relax. You must build up a habit of enjoying it instead of treating it as a necessary task. If you find that your body is a little bit sore the next day after practice, it is normal. However, if the soreness is significant, it implies you should proceed more slowly and more gradually.

To complete all of the exercises recommended, it will take about forty to fifty minutes. If you find that there are too many exercises, you may divide them into two or three groups and practice them alternatively. You may also select those exercises that are more beneficial to your needs. For example, if you have lower back pain, you may want to practice those exercises that focus on the lower back. If you have hip or knee joint problems, you may want to emphasize more on the hip and knee exercises. Naturally, you can always adjust the number of repetitions as well.

We will also introduce some important tui na and acupressure techniques in the next chapter. Again, if you find it takes too much time for you to do all of them each time, you may design your own schedule. For example, exercise in the morning, and massage before you go to sleep.

1-2. Meridian Qigong Exercises

Preparation

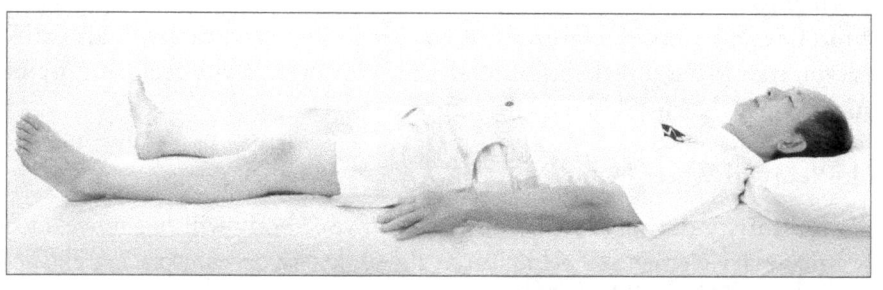

First lie facing upward, and completely relax. Remain calm throughout each exercise. Open your legs slightly, and place your arms comfortably beside your body. Inhale slowly and deeply, and then gently and slowly let the air out. Bring your attention to your body's feeling, and pay attention to the feeling in each area you are focusing on throughout the exercises. Remember, feeling is a language that allows your mind and body to communicate through the nervous system and qi (energy) circulation. If you are able to establish a deep feeling right at the beginning, you will have accomplished at least 50 percent of the effectiveness of these meridian qigong practices. Repeat this relaxed breathing at least three times.

Facing Upward

Arms/Legs (臂/腿)

1. Extend and Squeeze Fingers/Toes (Arms Straight Upward) 張指/張趾與 握拳/握趾 (上伸臂) 停 10 妙，重複2次

These exercises will lead the qi from the twelve qi channels, which are connected to the twelve internal organs, to your extremities. This is the first step to enliven and open the channels and improve your qi circulation right away.

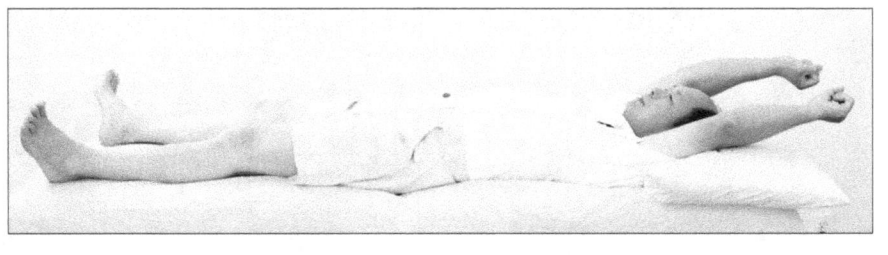

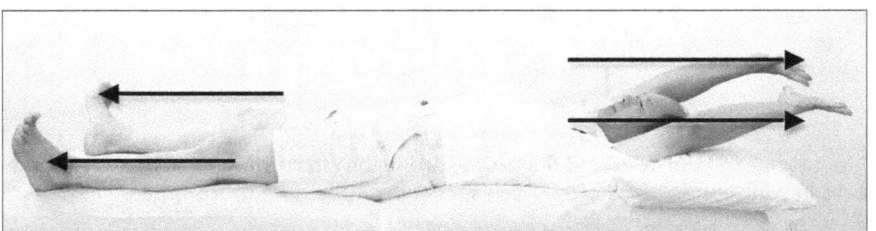

Extend both arms upward.

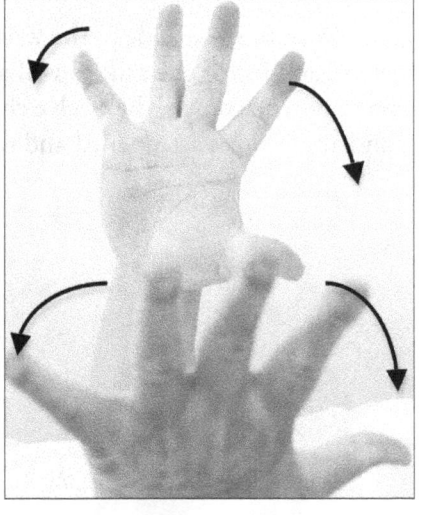 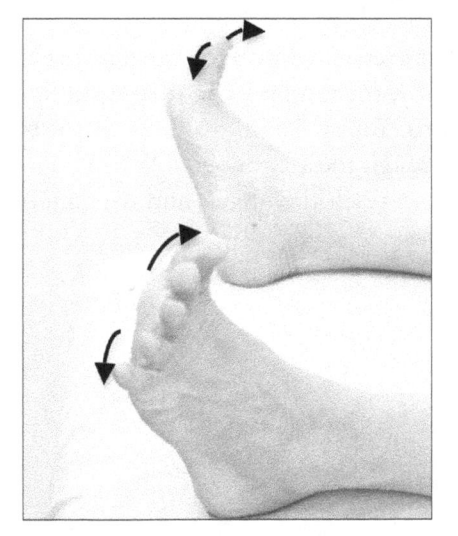

Open and stretch your toes and fingers as far as you can for ten seconds.

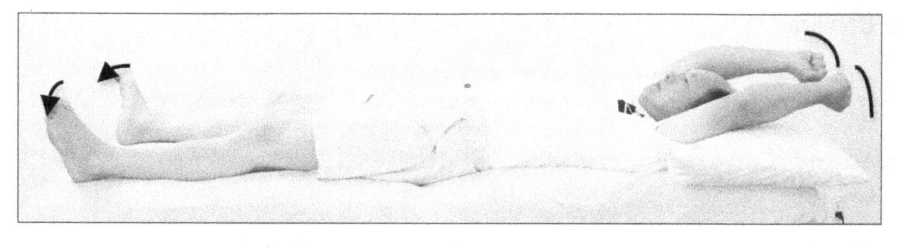

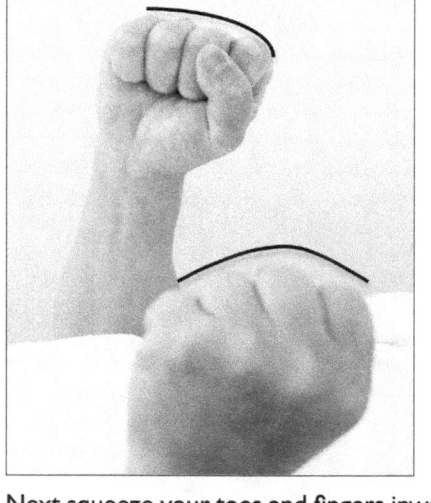
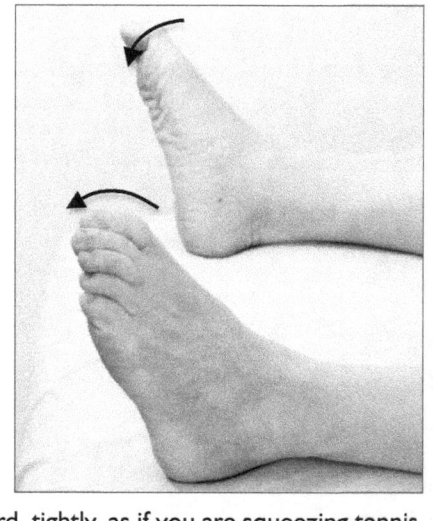

Next squeeze your toes and fingers inward, tightly, as if you are squeezing tennis balls in your hands, and hold for ten seconds. Repeat two more times.

2. Stretch Wrists/Ankles (Palms Facing Each Other) (拔腕/提足) (對掌) (手胸前) 停 **10** 妙，重複**2**次

This exercise will stretch the tendons and ligaments on the front side of the wrist area. Naturally, the tendons (Achilles) and ligaments on backside of the ankles will also be stretched. Your wrists and ankles are the two most important joints. The twelve channels pass through these two joints. When your wrist and ankle joints are opened and relaxed, the qi can reach the fingers and toes smoothly.

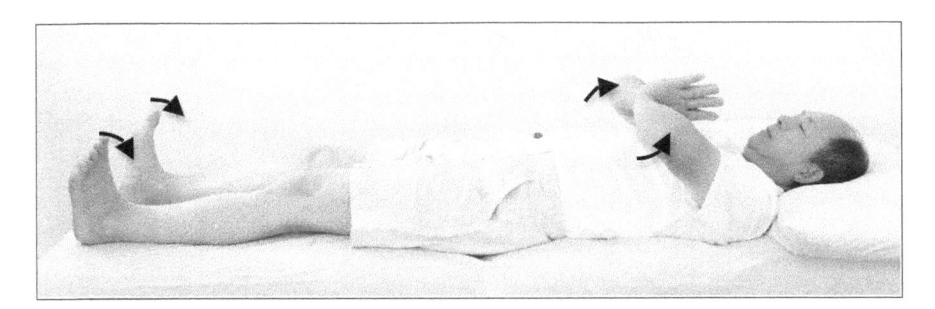

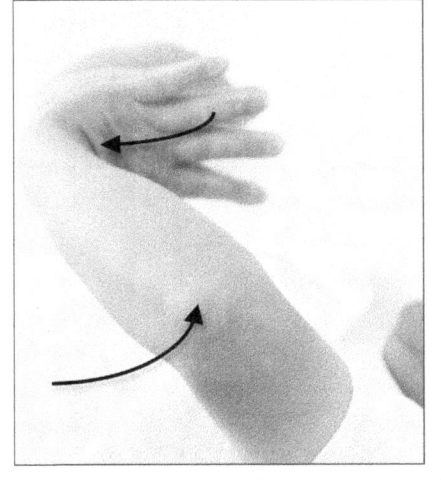 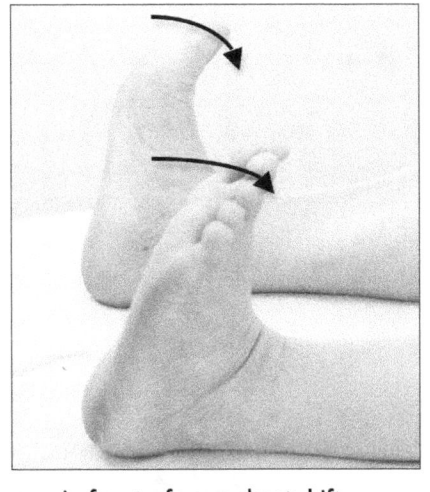

Face your palms together, aligning the fingers, in front of your chest. Lift up your elbows so the wrists are stretched backward. While you are doing so, also lift up your feet and bend them toward the shins. Stay in this position for ten seconds and then relax for five seconds. Repeat two more times.

3. Stretch Wrists/Ankles (Back of Hands Facing Each Other) (拔腕/伸足) (背掌) 停 10 妙，重複2次

This exercise is opposite of the previous one. You're stretching the backside of your wrists and also the front side of your ankles.

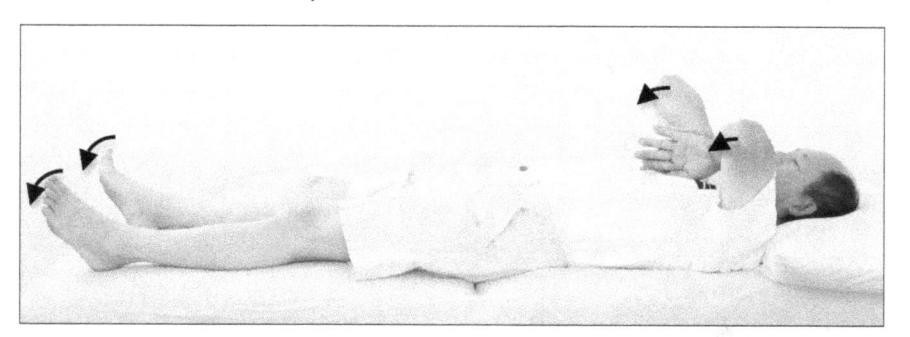

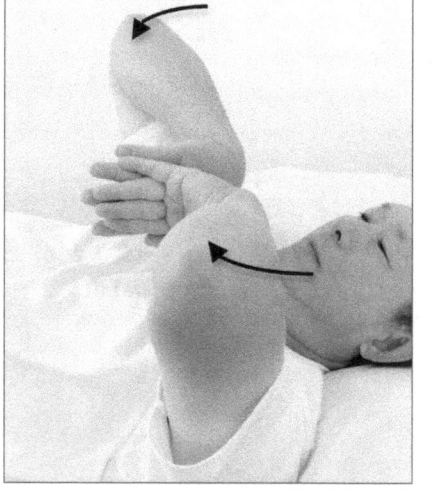

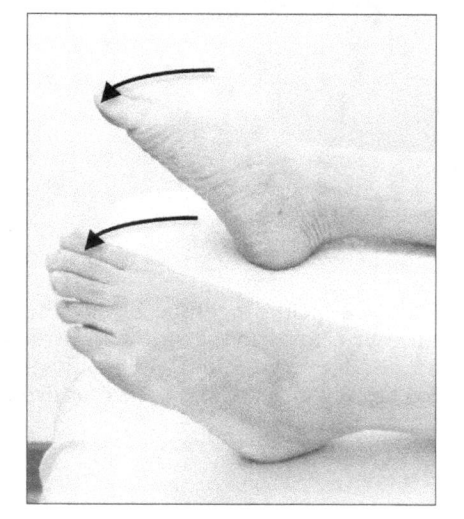

Face the back of your hands together with fingers aligned. Then lower your elbows to stretch the backside of your wrists. While you are doing so, extend your toes downward and stretch the front of your ankle joints. Stay in this position for ten seconds and then relax for five seconds. Repeat two more times.

4. Twist Wrists/Ankles (Outward) (拔腕/張足) (對掌扭擠) 停 10 妙，重複2次

This exercise stretches the sides of the wrists and ankles with a twisting action.

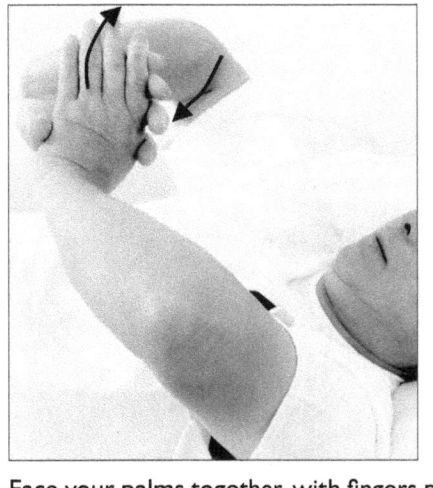 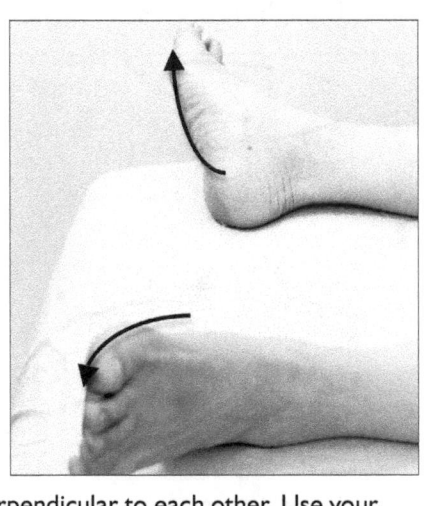

Face your palms together, with fingers perpendicular to each other. Use your right hand's pinky finger to press the index finger area of the left hand while using the left hand's index finger area to press the right hand's pinky finger. This will create a twisting of both wrists using reversed angles. While you are doing this, extend your toes outward and stretch your ankles outward. Stay in this position for ten seconds and then relax for five seconds. Repeat two more times.

5. Twist Wrists/Ankles (Inward) 拔腕/扣足) (換邊對掌扭擠) 停 10 妙，重複2次

This exercise is the reverse of the previous one.

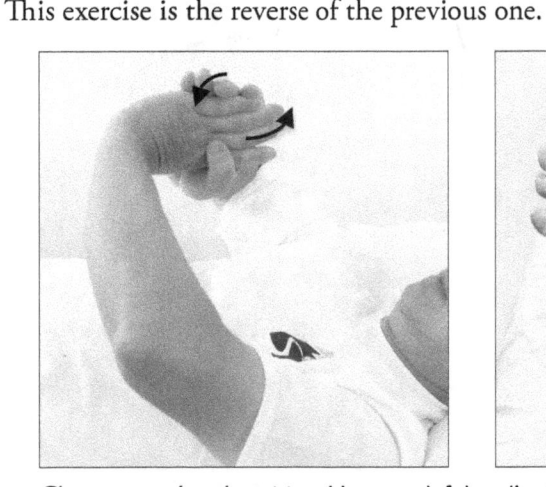 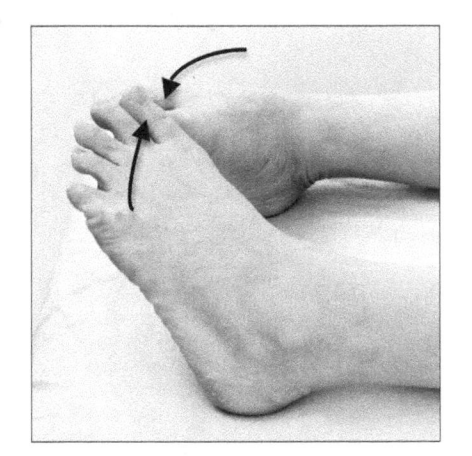

Change your hand position. Use your left hand's pinky finger area to press the index finger area of right hand and vice versa. While you are doing so, turn your toes inward and stretch your ankles inward. Stay in this position for ten seconds and then relax for five seconds. Repeat two more times.

6. Circle Wrists/Ankles (Outward Turning) (轉腕/轉踝) (外轉) **30** 次

This exercise will loosen up the wrist and ankle joints and open the twelve qi channels passing through these areas.

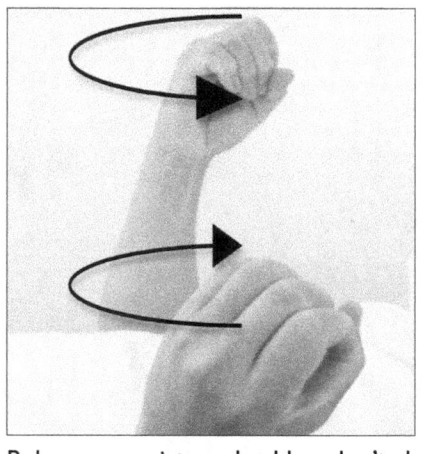 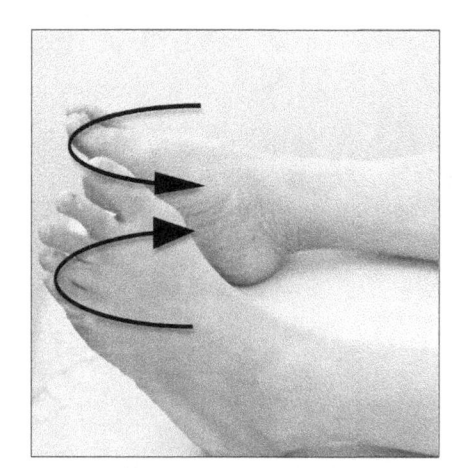

Relax your wrists and ankles; don't clench. Make circular motions with your hands and feet outward (i.e., right hand/foot clockwise and left hand/foot counterclockwise). Circle thirty times.

7. Circle Wrists/Ankles (Inward Turning) (轉腕/轉踝) (內轉) **30** 次

This exercise reverses the circular direction of the previous exercise and is part of loosening the wrist and ankle joints.

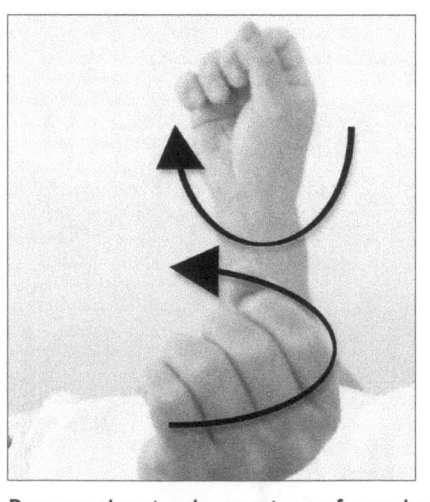 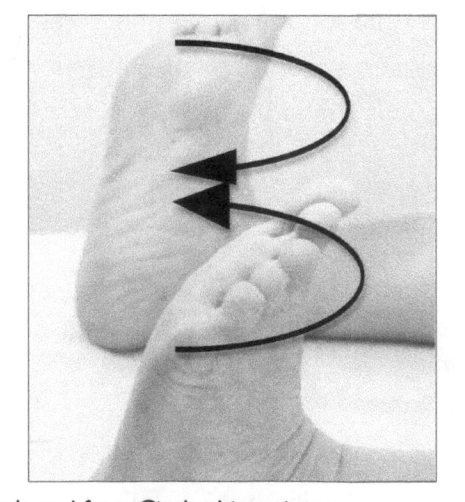

Reverse the circular motions of your hands and feet. Circle thirty times.

8. Sway Arms/Legs (晃臂/晃腿) (左右微晃) 30 次

This exercise will loosen up the muscles/tendons of the legs and arms and allow them to relax. Consequently, the qi channels will be opened for improved circulation.

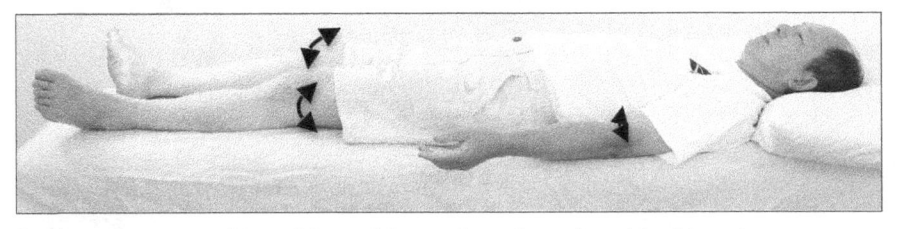

Sway your arms and legs side to side gently and comfortably thirty times.

9. Lift Forearms and Knees (提前臂/提膝) (易邊) 30 次

This exercise will loosen up the elbow and knee joints and allow qi to circulate smoothly in these joints.

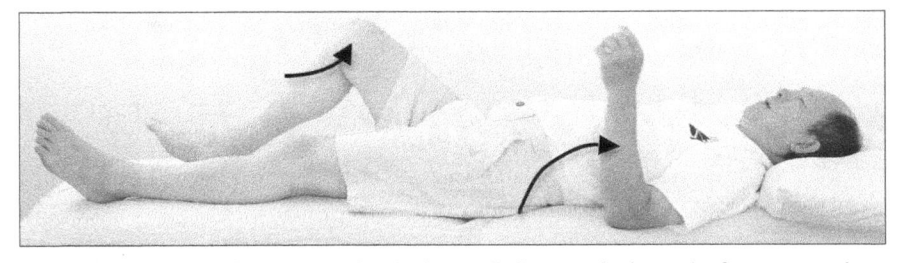

Gently lift your left forearm and right knee. Follow with the right forearm and left knee for thirty repetitions (fifteen times each side).

10. Lift Arms and Legs (提上臂/提腿) (彎肘) 30 次

This exercise will loosen up the shoulder and hip joints and allow qi to circulate smoothly in these areas. Your shoulders and hips are two of the most important qi junctions (joints) that connect the qi channels from the limbs to the torso.

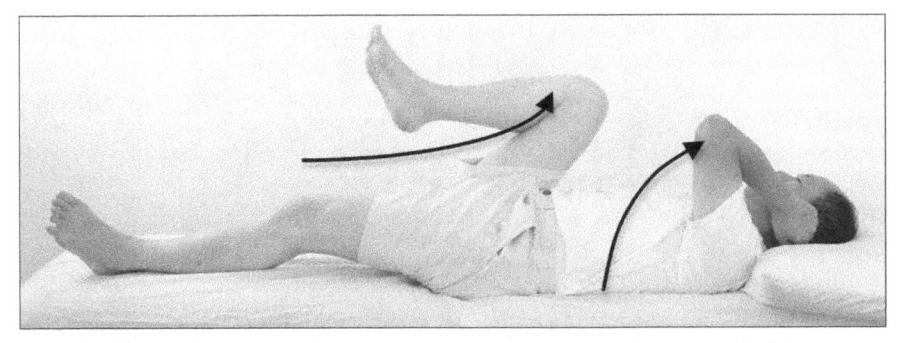

Lift your left arm and right leg gently. Follow with the right arm and left leg for thirty repetitions (fifteen times each side).

11. Close Arms/Knees Inward and Open Them Outward (展臂/展腿) (彎小腿) (雙展) 30 次

Because all the muscles/tendons on the hip joints connect to the lower back, this exercise will begin to loosen up the lower back area.

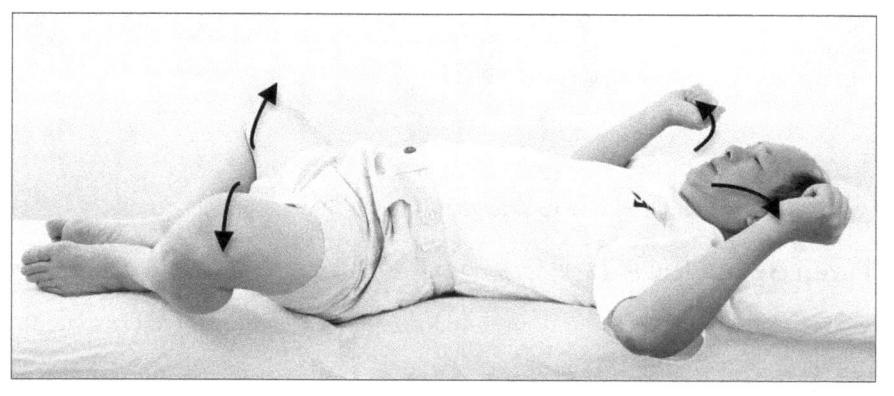

Bend both elbows and knees and then swing them inward and outward like a butterfly thirty times (fifteen times each direction).

12. Open and Close Single Arm/Knee (展臂/展腿) (彎小腿) (單展) 30 次

This exercise will begin to loosen the upper back area.

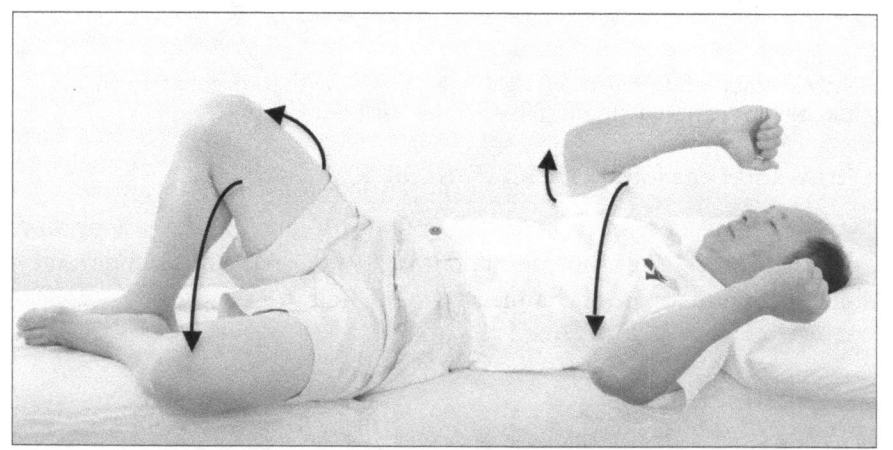

Keep your arms and legs bent. Open and close your arm and leg on one side and then the other side thirty times (fifteen times each side).

13. Swing Arms and Legs Opposite Sides (展臂/展腿) (並腿) (臂腿異向) 30 次

This torso-twisting exercise will open and loosen up all the muscles/tendons in your torso that connect to the hips.

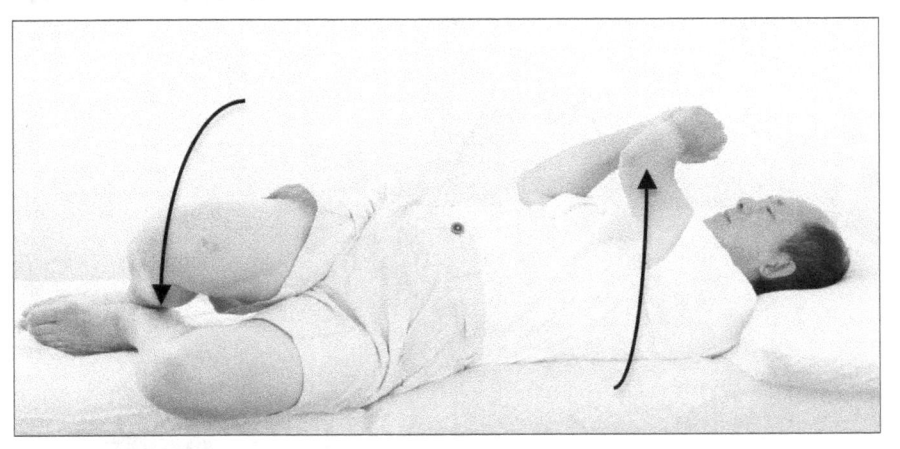

Close your arms and legs and swing them in the opposite direction thirty times (fifteen times each side).

Waist/Hips

14. Embrace Knees and Swing (Apanasana) (抱膝左右晃) 30次

This exercise will begin to stretch the torso and loosen it up, especially the lower back area.

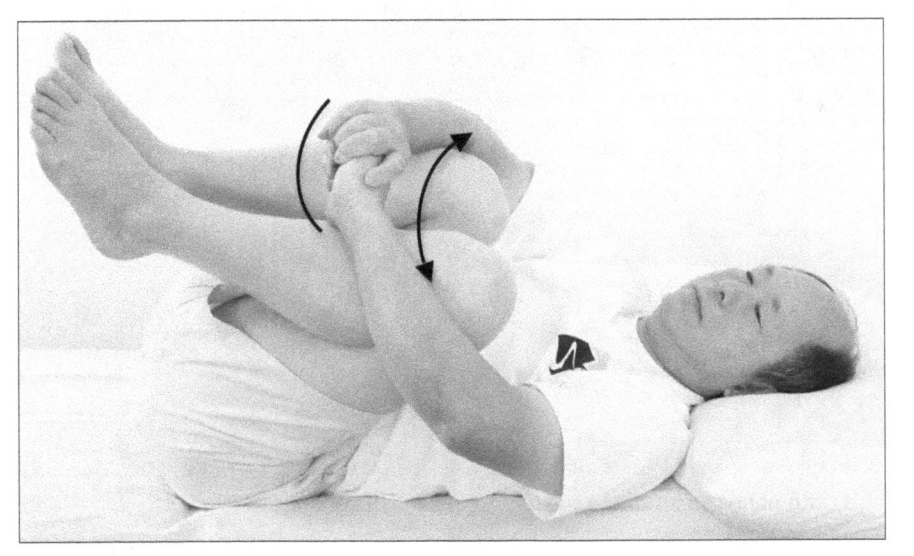

Use both arms to embrace the knees or upper shin area and then swing them from side to side thirty times.

15. Pull Legs and Swing (Ananda Balasana) (拉腿左右晃) 30次

This exercise will enhance the stretching.

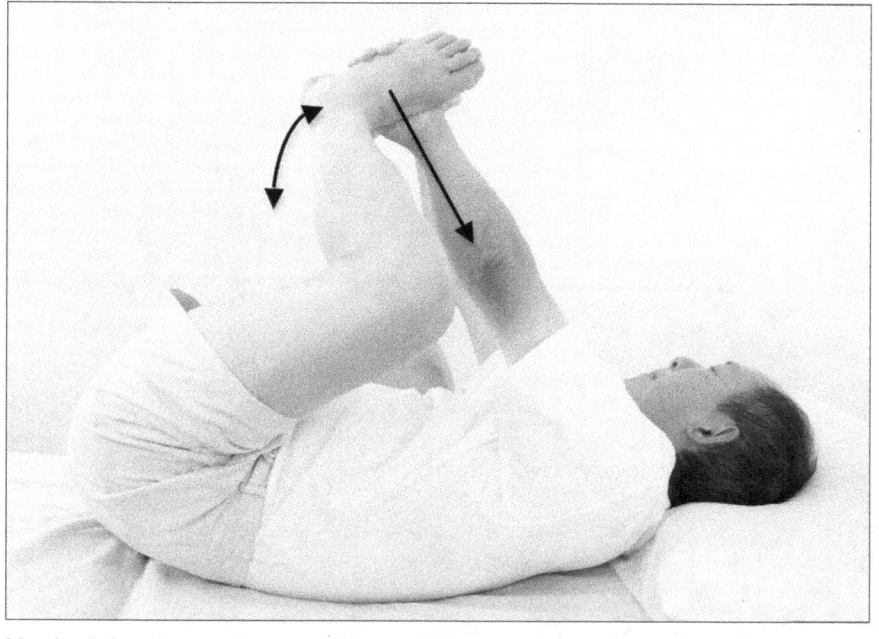

Use both hands to pull your legs upward around the ankle areas and then swing from side to side thirty times.

16. Embrace, Open, and Press Single Leg (Supta Kaptasana, Modified)

(單腿盤拉) (抱、張、壓) 30 秒

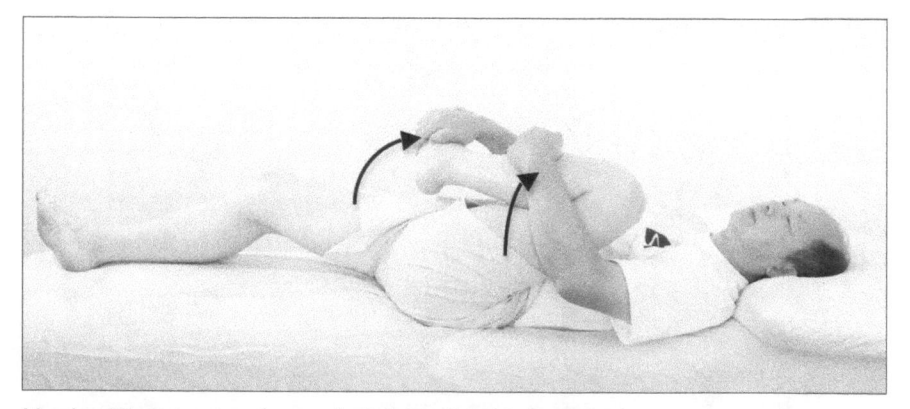

Use both hands to embrace the left leg for thirty seconds.

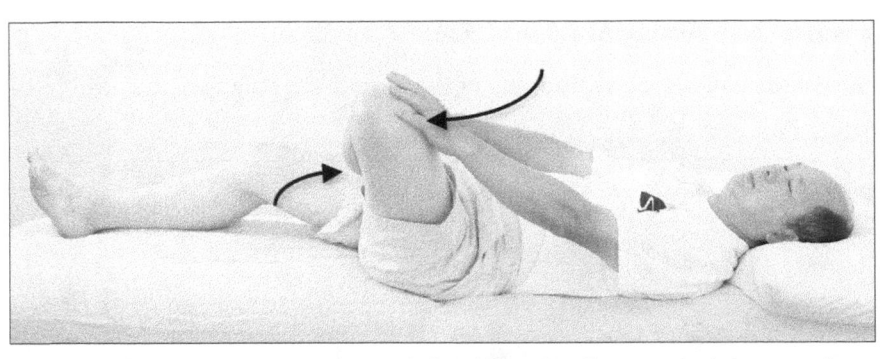

Next use the right hand to grab your left ankle and pull upward while using the left hand to push the left knee downward for thirty seconds.

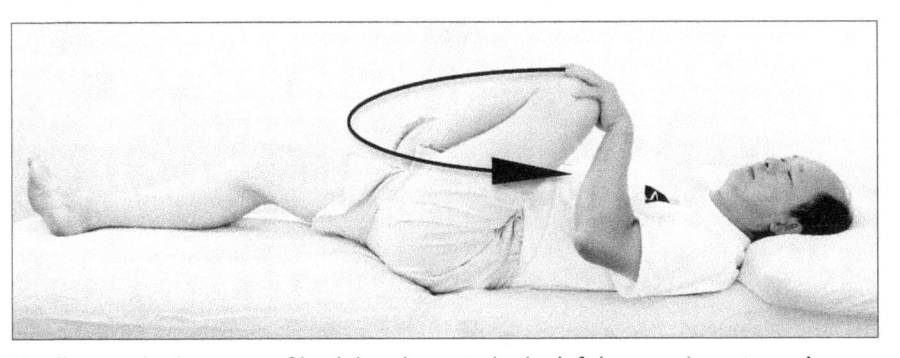

Finally, use the leverage of both hands to circle the left leg ten times in each direction. Switch to the other leg, and repeat the same process.

Waist/Torso

17. Sway Waist/Torso (晃腰/軀幹) (左右) 30 次

After the stretching exercises, this exercise will further release tension.

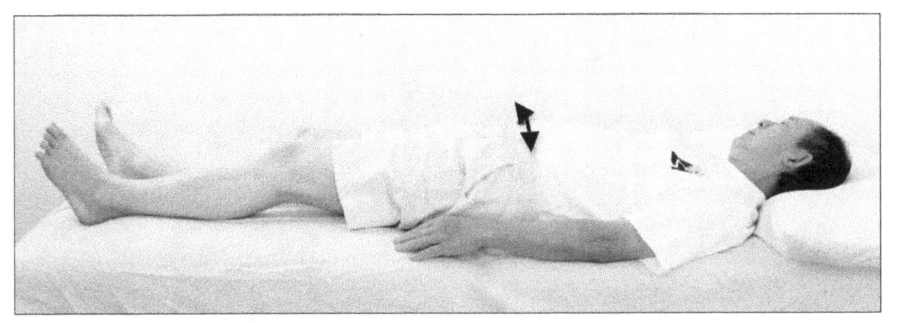

Keep your legs straight with both arms comfortably beside your torso. Sway your torso, especially your waist area, side to side thirty times.

18. Lift Waist (Setu Asana, Moving) (提腰) (彎膝) 30 次

This exercise begins the conditioning of the lower back structure including ligaments, muscles, and tendons.

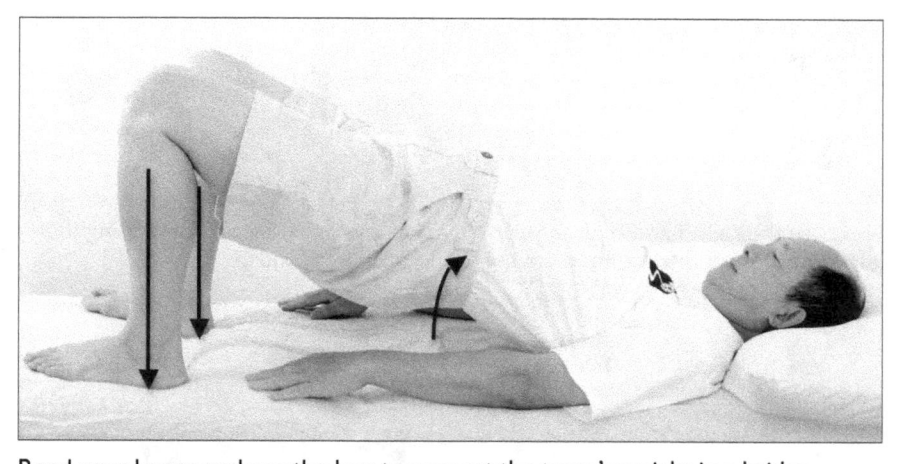

Bend your knees and use the legs to support the torso's weight in a bridge posture. Lift your waist up and down thirty times.

19. Circle Waist (Setu Asana, Circling) (腰繞圈) (彎膝) 每邊 20 次

This exercise continues to condition the lower back area. If you find this conditioning exercise and the lift-waist exercise too difficult, reduce the number of repetitions. Be careful not to harm your lower back. Listen to your body, and gradually increase the number of comfortable repetitions. Good soreness and comfortable pain are appropriate ways of conditioning. If the pain is too significant and soreness is too severe, it will only cause tightness and make the qi circulation more stagnant.

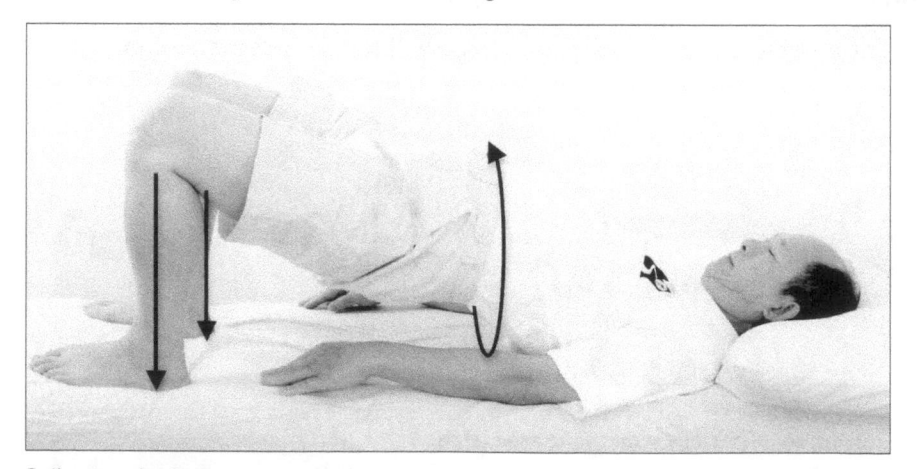

Still using the legs to support the lower back, circle the waist area clockwise twenty times and then reverse the direction for another twenty times.

20. Tighten and Loosen Hips/Perineum (Mula Bandha) (緊鬆胯部/穀道) 30次

This exercise is for the muscles/tendons that connect the hips and anus muscles. The most important aspect of this practice is to exercise your huiyin (會陰, CV-1) (perineum) cavity. It is well known in Chinese medicine and qigong that the huiyin cavity is the crucial key acupoint that controls the qi's circulation in and out of the central body. This cavity acts as the piston of the pump for your main energy center, known as the lower real dan tian (下真丹田). When it is pushed out, the qi in the body is released, and when it is held upward, the qi stays in the central body. Training the muscles in this area will allow you to effectively control this cavity.

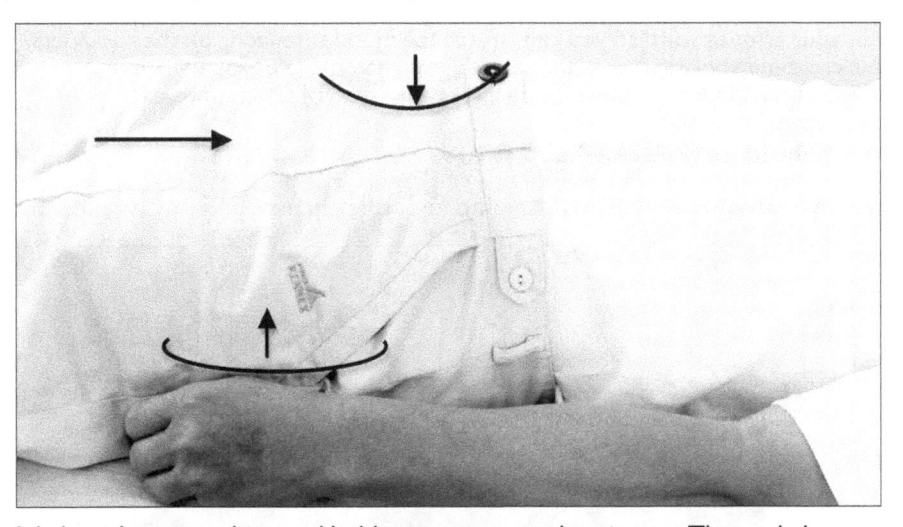

Inhale, tighten your hips, and hold up your anus and perineum. Then exhale, relax your hips, and gently push your anus out for thirty repetitions.

21. Shoulders/Torso/Neck Lift Torso and Shoulder from Side to Side (Arms Beside Torso) (提軀幹/肩膀) (垂臂) 左右各 10 次

This exercise will loosen up the torso and exercise the muscles and tendons connecting to the lower back.

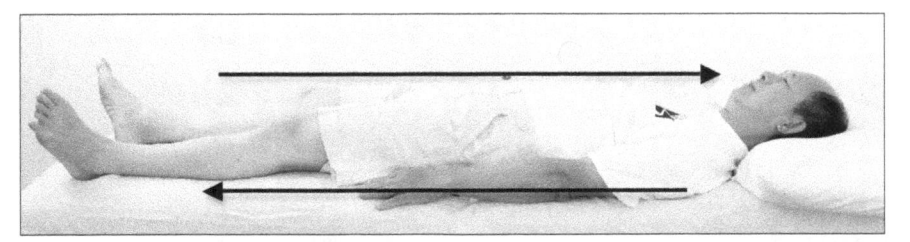

Place both arms comfortably beside your torso. Raise your right shoulder and torso and then raise the left side, ten times each side.

22. Lift Torso and Shoulder from Side to Side (Arms Upward)
(提軀幹/肩膀) (上伸臂) 左右各**10**次

This exercise enhances the stretching of the torso muscles connecting to the lower back.

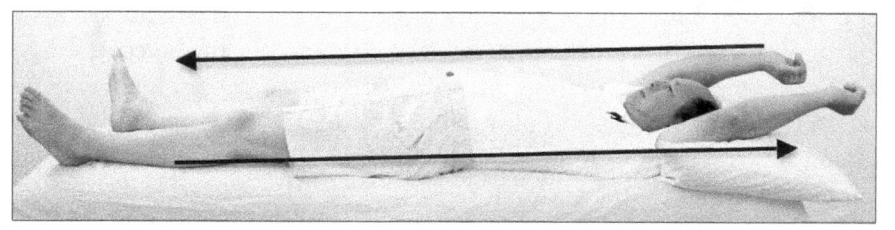

Lift your arms upward so you can stretch the muscles/tendons on the shoulders.
Next extend your right arm and torso higher than the left to stretch your arm
and torso, and then lift the left side higher than the right, ten times each side.

23. Circle Shoulders (肩膀繞圈) 正反各**10**次

This exercise loosens up the shoulder joints and will help prevent many shoulder problems.

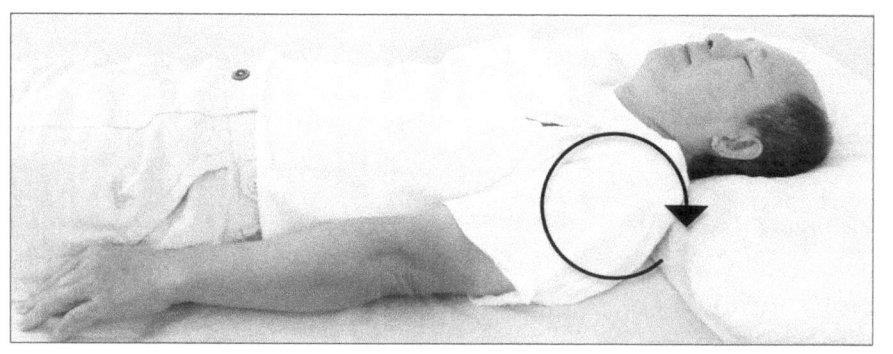

Place your arms beside your torso so they are comfortably situated. Circle one
shoulder ten times and then the other side ten times. When you circle them,
make sure the circles are as big as possible so the tendons and ligaments are
stretched. The direction of the circling is not important.

24. Stretch and Open Four Limbs (四肢分張) **20** 秒，重復一次

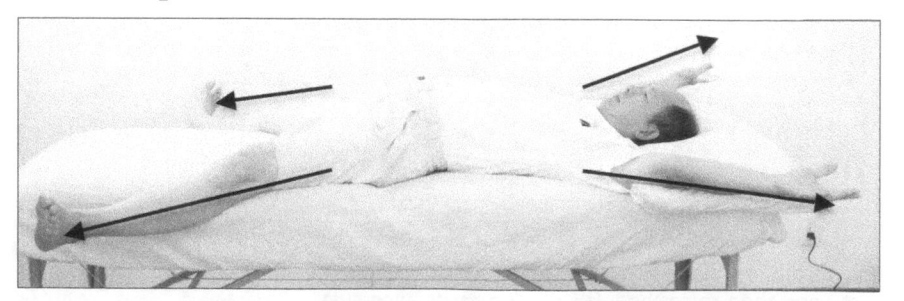

Open and extend your arms and legs as wide as possible. Stay in this stretched
position for twenty seconds. Relax for five seconds, and then repeat.

25. Stretch and Open Four Limbs (Opposite Sides) (左右開拔) 每邊2次，每次10妙

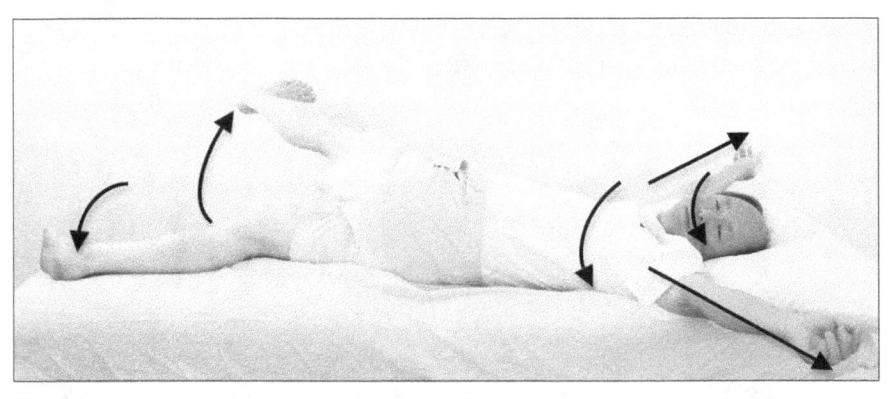

Keep both arms opened, and cross your legs so your torso is twisted and stretched. While you are twisting your torso, you should also turn your head to the opposite side so the neck can be stretched and you experience a full spinal twist. Stay in this position for ten seconds, and then switch the position of your legs to the opposite side and hold for another ten seconds. Repeat.

26. Turn the Head Left and Right (左右轉頭) 每邊10次

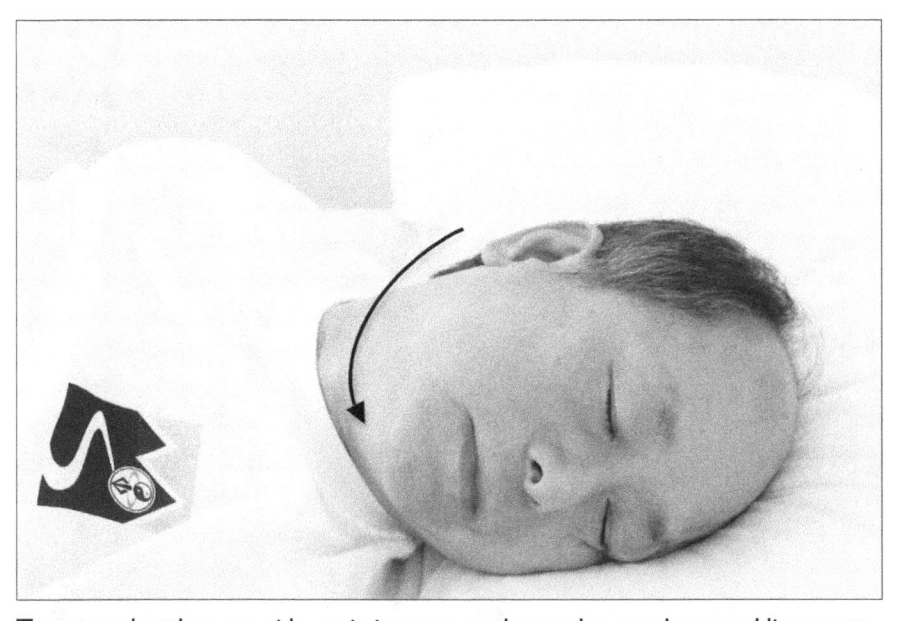

Turn your head to one side, twisting your neck muscles, tendons, and ligaments, and hold for three seconds. Change to the other side for another three seconds. Repeat ten times on each side.

27. Toss the Body Left and Right (左右翻身) 每邊10次

This exercise will loosen up the entire torso. If you find that this turning exercise makes you feel dizzy or nauseated, you should reduce the number of repetitions.

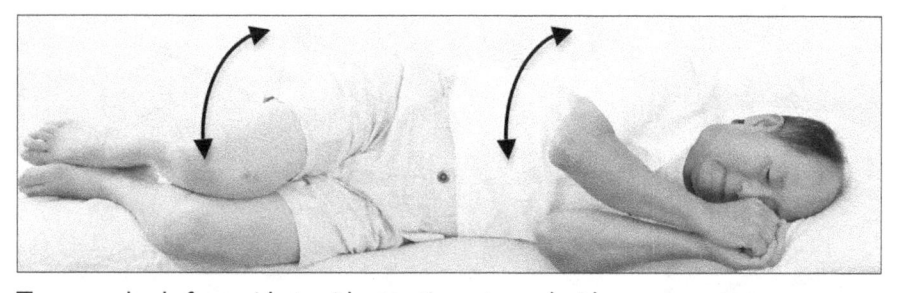

Toss your body from side to side, ten times to each side.

28. Sway the Body Sideways (側躺微晃) 每邊30 次

This exercise will relax the torso and allow qi to circulate smoothly. You'll find it can be very pleasant, like rocking yourself to sleep.

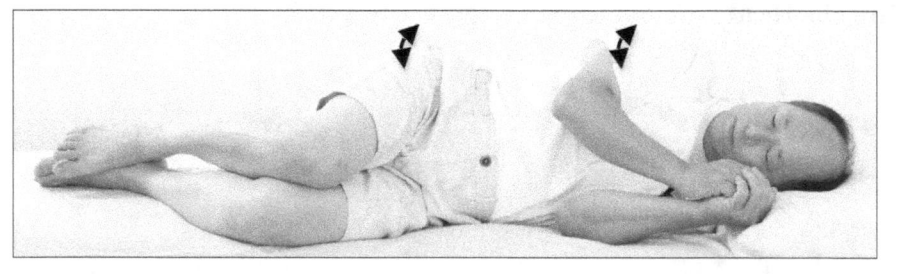

Turn your body to one side, and then rock and sway gently and lightly thirty times. Turn to the other side, and rock and sway again thirty times.

Facing Downward

29. Left and Right Sway the Body (左右晃身) (面朝下平身) 每邊30 次

This exercise will loosen up the back-muscle tension caused by facing upward.

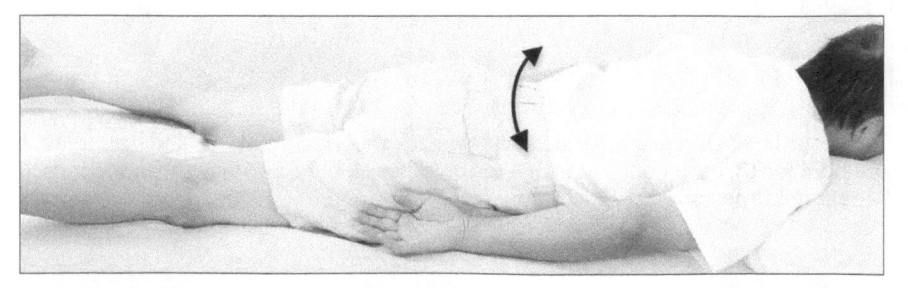

Turn your body, and lie facing downward. Swing your waist area left and right gently to loosen up the torso. Swing thirty times.

30. Sway Hips (臀左右晃) (跪式) 每邊30 次

This exercise will loosen up the lower back muscles.

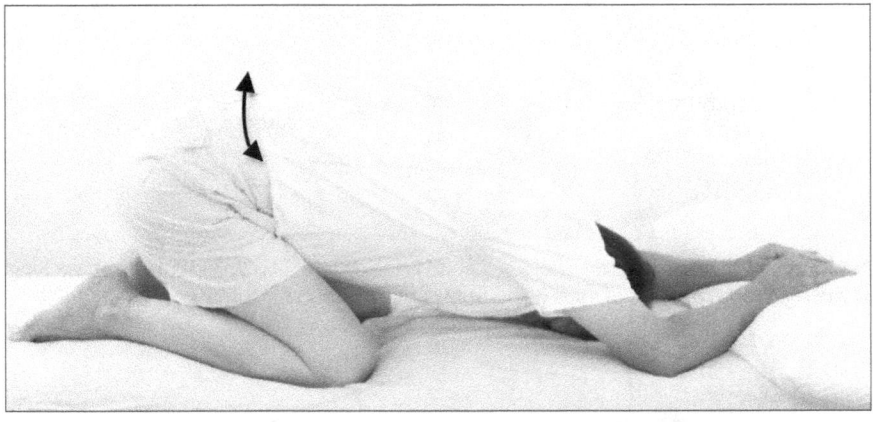

Pull your legs into a kneeling posture. Gently sway your hips from side to side thirty times.

31. Stretch the Torso—Forward, Left, and Right (跪拔上身) (前、左、右拔) 30 秒

This stretching exercise will open up tight back muscles.

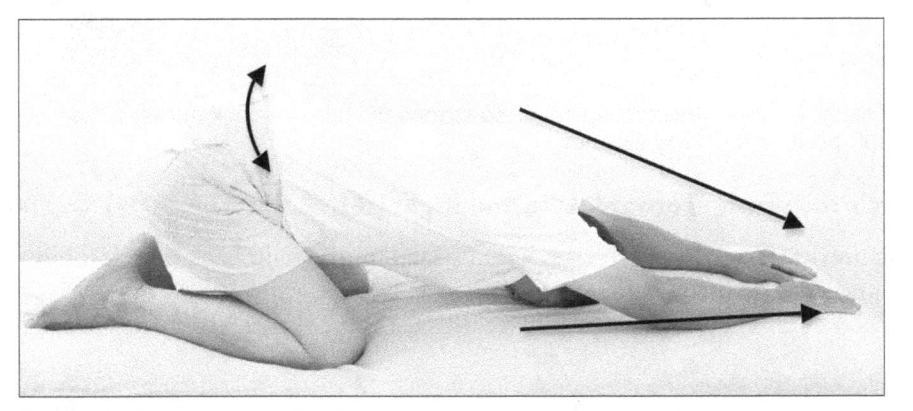

Extend both arms forward as far as you can so that the torso is stretched. Stay there for about thirty seconds. If you like, you may gently swing your hips from side to side while maintaining the stretch.

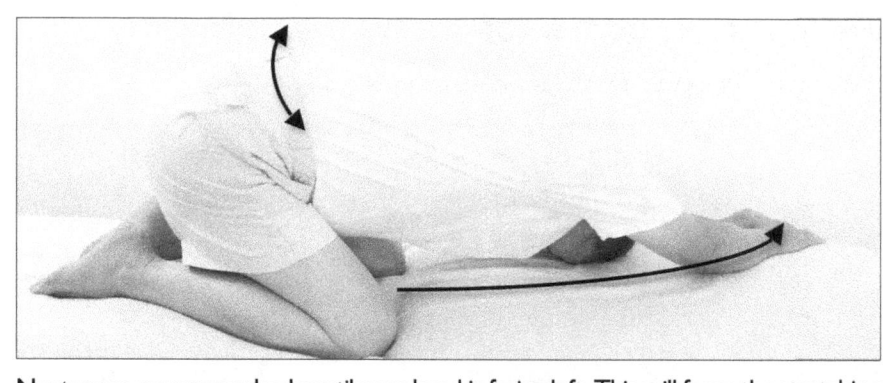

Next move your upper body until your head is facing left. This will focus the stretching in the right-side muscles of your back. Stay in this position for thirty seconds.

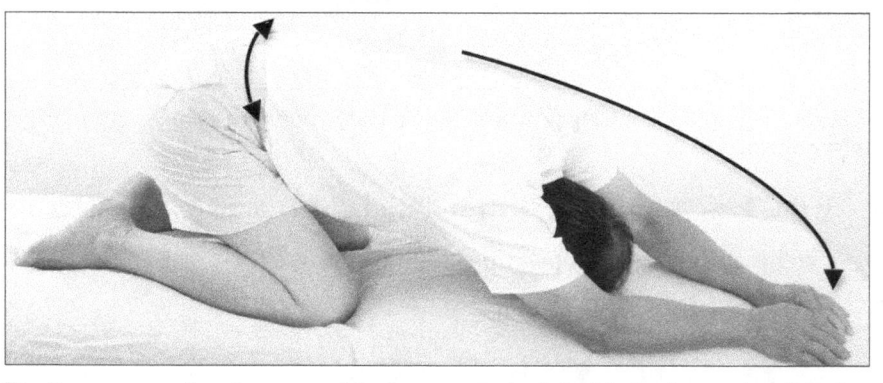

Finally, turn your head to your right to stretch the left-side back muscles. Stay in this position for thirty seconds.

32. Circle the Waist—Forward, Left, and Right (腰部繞圈) (前、左、右繞) 每邊30 次

The previous stretching exercises have opened up the tight back muscles. Now we go deeper and exercise the vertebrae.

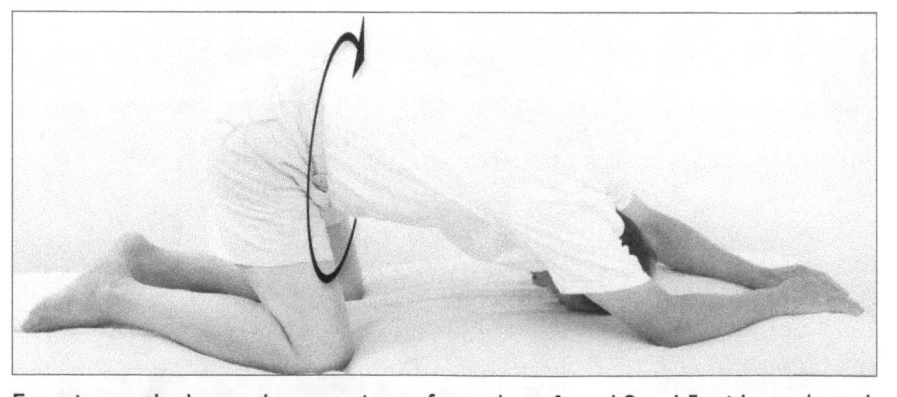

Focusing on the lower three sections of vertebrae from L2 to L5 with gentle and slow circular movements, circle thirty times, and then reverse the circling direction for another thirty times.

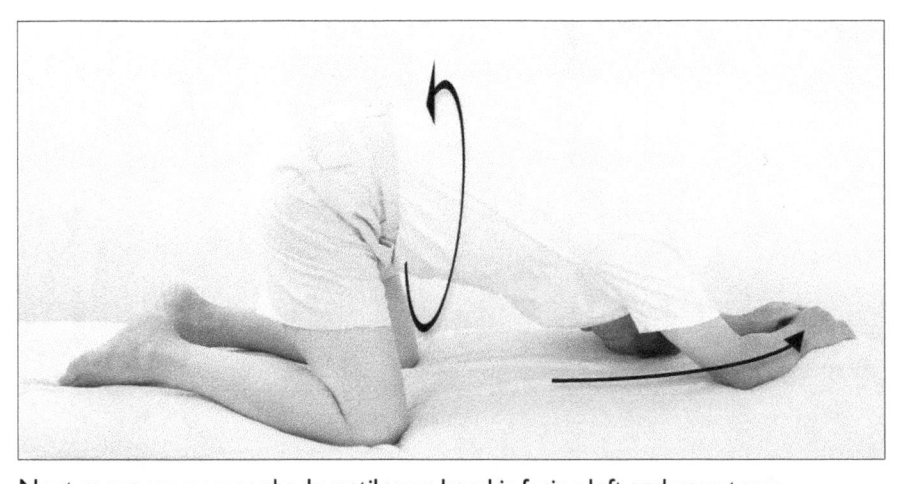

Next move your upper body until your head is facing left and your torso stretches to the left. Repeat the waist circular motion thirty times. Finally, change to the other side, and repeat the circular motion thirty times. Remember, you should focus the movement in the lower back.

33. Spine Waving (Marjari Asana) (脊椎波動) 每邊30 次

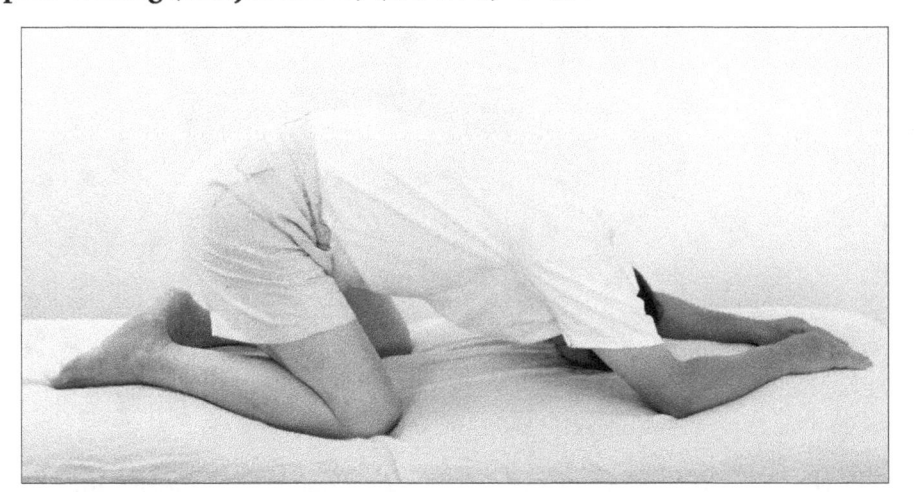

Move your upper body forward again with your elbows comfortably supporting the upper body and the head facing down.

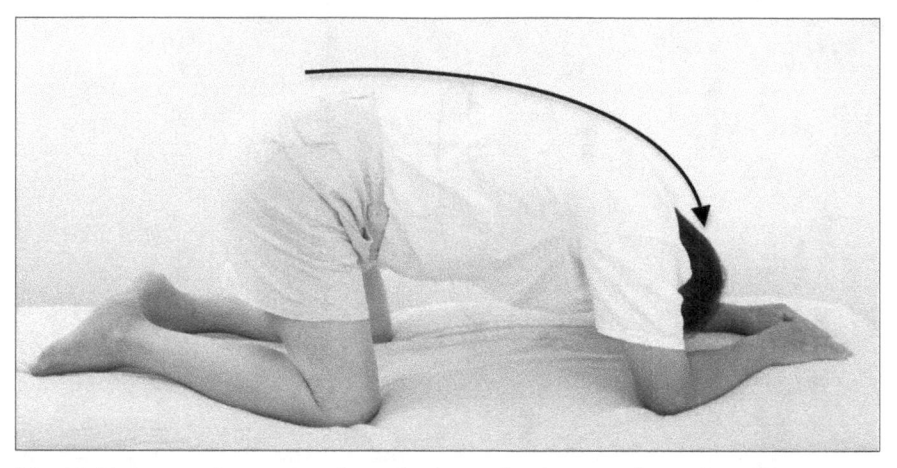

Next initiate a waving motion from the lower back upward, moving your vertebrae section by section. Repeat thirty times.

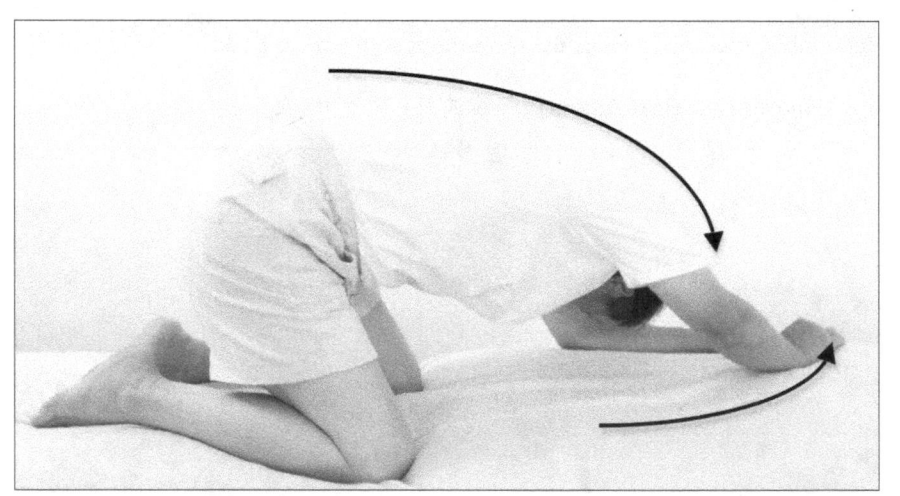

Then turn your upper body to the left and repeat the same spine-waving movement thirty times.

Finally, turn your body to your right, and repeat the same movement thirty times.

Recovery

If you decide to continue your practice to the full self-massage regimen, you may skip these recovery exercises and go straight to massage. Most of these exercises will be repeated in the massage chapter.

1. Massage the Abdomen Gently with Circular Motion (圈摩腹部)

After you finish your spine-waving movement, lie facing upward. Remember, you should feel comfortable. If you feel uncomfortable, you should stop massaging.

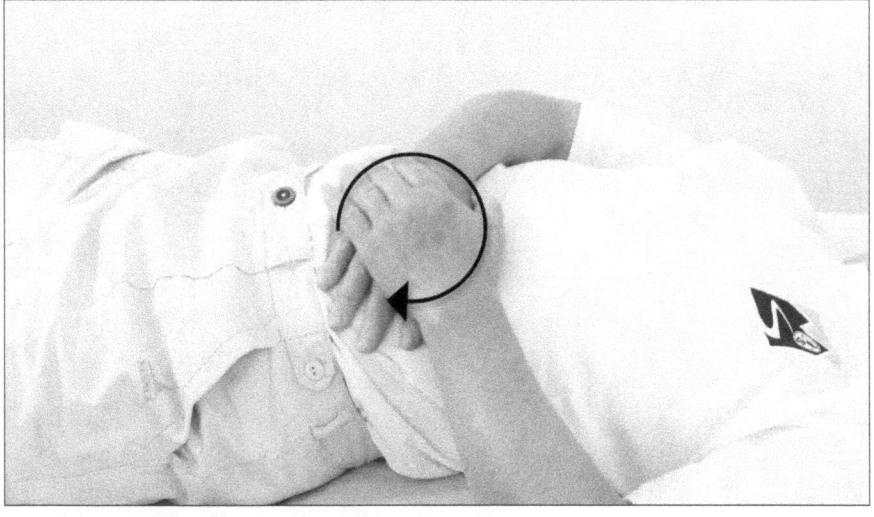

Use both hands to gently and comfortably massage the stomach and abdominal areas with a circular motion following the direction of the bowel system. In other words, starting from just above your belly button, circle your hands to your left, then down, then to your right, and around back to above your belly button. Massaging in this direction smooths the qi circulation. If you reverse the direction, you may create stagnation in the circulation, and that may cause constipation. You should massage in circles until a warm feeling gets deeper and deeper.

2. Massage the Inner Hip Joints (搓摩胯部)

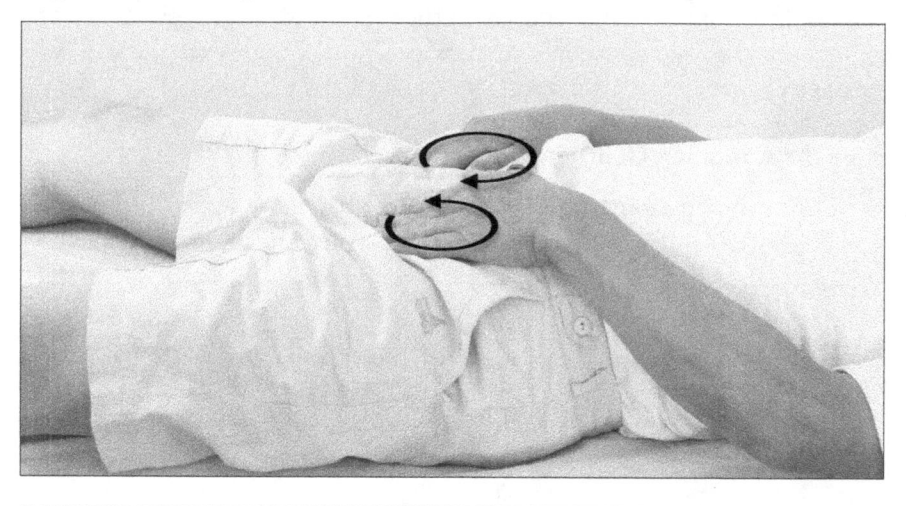

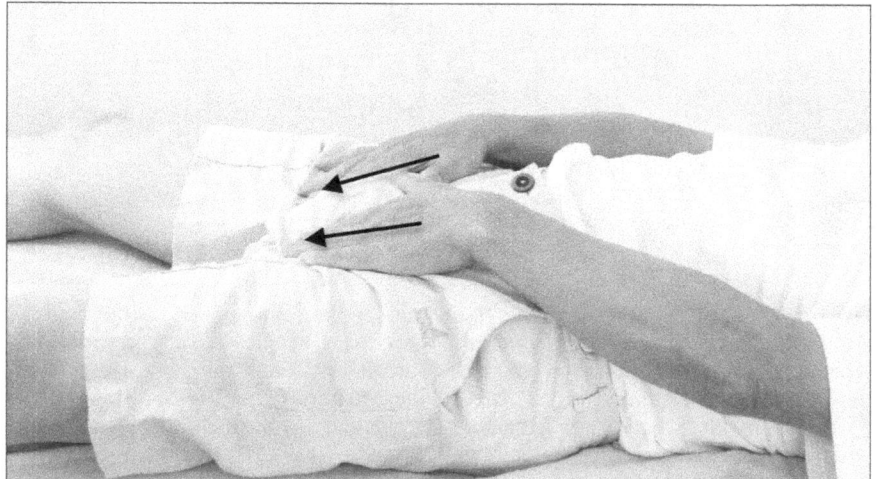

Next extend your massage to the lower abdominal area and groin area. Gently massage the entire area for a couple of minutes, and then gently slide downward to the sides of the groin and inner hips. Massage for three to five minutes.

3. Massage Testicles/Ovaries (按摩睪丸/卵巢) and Pressing Huiyin (指點會陰)

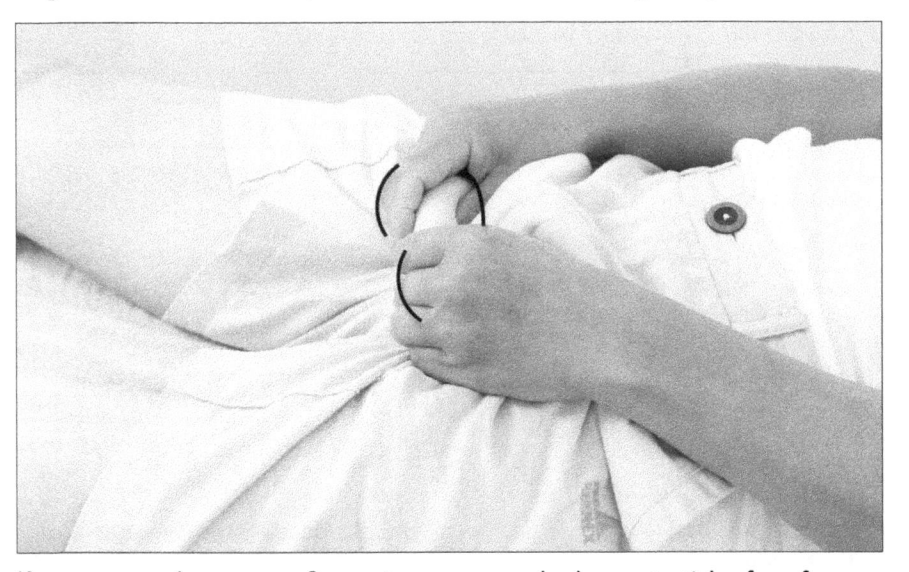

If you are a male, use your fingers to massage and rub your testicles for a few minutes. If you massage too much and feel uncomfortable, you should stop.

If you are a female, you may massage the ovary areas for a few minutes. Again, if you feel uncomfortable, you should stop.

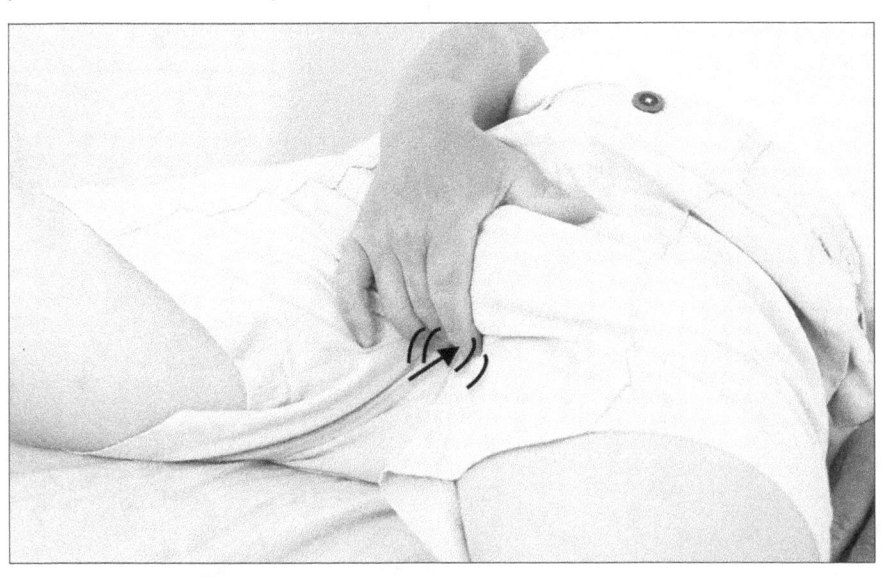

After massaging, use your middle finger to press the perineum/huiyin (CV-1) (會陰) cavity and gently circle rub ten times in each direction to loosen the muscle. This massage allows your qi to move more freely. While you are massaging the perineum/huiyin, you should gently hold up your anus.

4. Abdominal Deep Breathing (小腹順息)

This is a relaxing "Buddhist" breath.

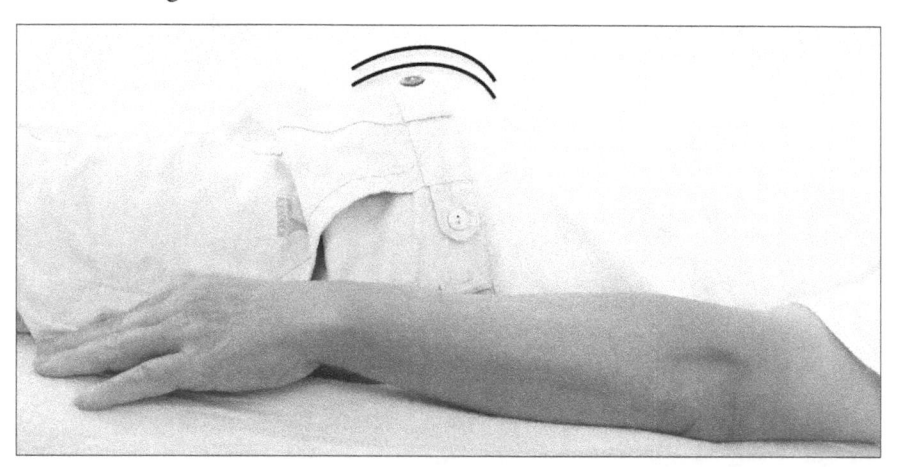

Place both arms beside your body and relax. Breathe deeply and move your abdomen with each breath. When you inhale, you should expand your abdomen and gently push out your anus; when you exhale, you should withdraw your abdomen and gently pull in your anus. Repeat the breathing for three to five minutes.

5. Circle the Tongue to Generate Saliva (赤龍攪津)

End the sequence by circling the tongue.

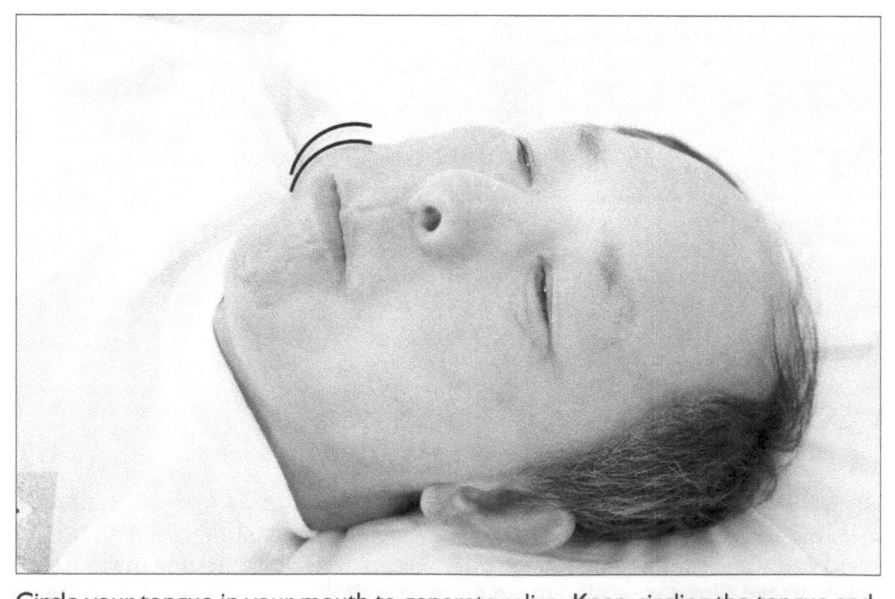

Circle your tongue in your mouth to generate saliva. Keep circling the tongue and collect saliva until the mouth is full. Then divide the saliva into three gulps, and swallow it while breathing deeply. If you have time, you should repeat two more times.

Chapter 2: Self-Massage—Tui Na and Dian Xue

2-1. Introduction

Tui (推) means "push," and na (拿) means "grab." Therefore, tui na massage means the massage focused on techniques of pushing and grabbing. Tui na is one of the main massage techniques developed in China. Tui na massage has commonly been used for injury treatments and also infant sicknesses. From tui na, the cells can be stimulated to a higher energized state, and the irregular qi circulation can be corrected.

Dian (點) means "pointing," and xue (穴) means "cavity." Dian xue massage is also called acupressure. By applying pressure to some acupuncture cavities, the qi circulation in the twelve primary channels (meridians) can be manipulated. Consequently, many sicknesses can be prevented or healed.

Traditionally, it would take at least ten years of learning and practicing for a tui na and dian xue masseur or masseuse to reach a professional level and become a healer. However, there are many cavities and techniques you can use for basic health prevention or even some level of healing that do not require long-term professional training.

Professional tui na and dian xue masseurs must know approximately 108 cavities of the more than seven hundred cavities in the body. Through these cavities, without using needles, the qi circulating in the primary qi channels can be manipulated and improved. To learn massage, the first step is self-massage. Through your experience with self-massage, you will see the accuracy of pushing, grabbing, and cavity press. The most important aspect of all is to develop the feeling of the power and its penetration. This feeling is a crucial key in becoming a good masseur. However, if you wish to become a professional tui na and dian xue masseur or masseuse, you still need to find a professional school or experienced massage doctor to guide you to the depth of this massage art.

This chapter will cover only a small portion of tui na and dian xue massage techniques. Through self-massage you will be able to feel and experience the effectiveness of these massages. When training yourself, it can be very beneficial to be familiar with some important cavities and their related illnesses. Most important of all, by massaging these cavities often, you will be able to maintain your health.

The best time to practice these massage techniques is right after waking up. This is because when you are sleeping, your physical body is relaxing and not in action, and the qi circulation slows down. Early morning massage will help you enhance the qi circulation and energize yourself. The second best time is right before sleeping. Through massaging these cavities, you are able to open up the qi channels that can be stagnant after a whole day's activities. The only disadvantage to self-massage is you will not be able to easily massage your own back area where there are many important crucial cavities for health maintenance.

It takes about twenty minutes to massage yourself each time. However, if you don't have too much time, then you may massage every other day. Naturally, you may also massage these cavities whenever you wish.

In this chapter we will introduce self-massage divided into five sections: I. Head and Neck; II. Chest and Abdomen; III. Lower Back and Hips (Facing Upward); IV. Lower Back and Hips (Facing Sideways); and V. Limbs.

2-2. Tui Na and Dian Xue Self-Massage

Self-massage has many benefits and advantages. Once you understand these benefits, you will realize that your health is in your hands, and you don't have to rely on other people's help.

Benefits and Advantages of Self-Massage

1. You can massage yourself any time and any place. You don't have to take a masseuse with you or find one when you need one.

2. Because you are the one massaging yourself, you have control over the feeling and power used. Through feeling, you always know how much power is needed and how effective it will be for you. When you receive a massage from someone other than a highly professional masseur or masseuse, oftentimes the power used does not match the desired or ideal pressure.

3. From self-massage, you will be familiar with many massage techniques and the correct feeling. Not only that, the knowledge you will gain through understanding the concept and experimenting will offer you a lifetime of benefits.

Disadvantages of Self-Massage

1. You cannot massage your upper back between the shoulder blades, and the upper back is considered one of the major areas that need to be massaged. This is because the upper back area is the key junction area where your energy is communicating between the head, shoulders, and lower torso.

2. Because you need to use physical movement to massage yourself, there is more tension, both mentally and physically.

Before you get involved in the practice of this chapter, there are a few general rules and tips you should be aware of.

General Rules

1. The number of repetitions or the duration of massage suggested is adjustable because everyone has different sensitivity and body structure. You should experience it, and gradually adjust it for yourself.

2. If you find your time is limited, you may alternate the qigong exercises and massages daily. Naturally, if you have time, it will be better if you can do qigong exercises first, followed by massage. You can also choose to do one in the morning and the other in the evening.

3. Dian xue (cavity press) is able to stimulate the deep areas of the body so the qi circulation in primary channels (meridians) can be regulated. In addition, through cavity press, the stagnant qi accumulated in the cavity areas can be brought to the surface. This will help to release the qi knots or stagnation. Then, if you follow with circular rubbing, you will be able to spread the qi to the wider area on the surface. Finally, use tui na to push the qi away from the stimulated area. Usually, for releasing the qi, the direction of pushing is from top to the lower part of the body and from center of the body to the sides, torso, or the limbs.

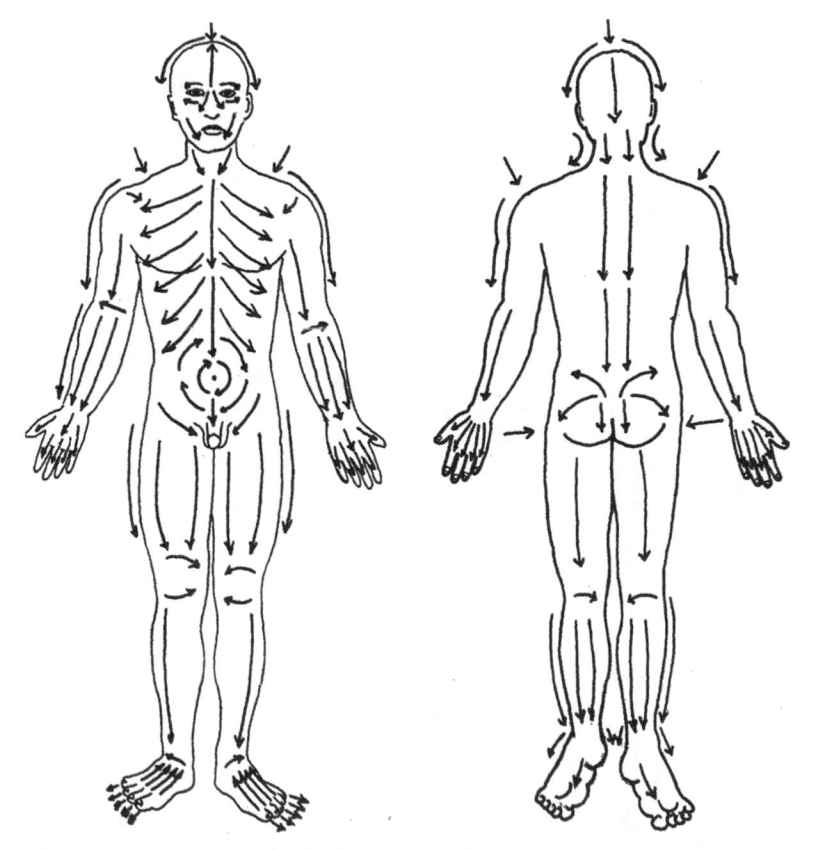

Massage pathways on the body in general qigong massage.

4. There are two common cavity-stimulation techniques: press vibrating and rubbing with circular motion. When you press and vibrate, usually you use a sharper area of your fingers, such as the tip of the thumb or toes, so the power can be more penetrating.

Good stimulation is about ten seconds. After that, allow the muscle tissue to relax for a few seconds, and then stimulate again. Then you should rub the area with a softer part of your fingers or foot. The rubbing massage is able to bring the stagnant qi from deep within the body to the surface. Not only that, it can also help to spread the qi to a wider area and allow the body to naturally and more easily disperse it.

5. Fingernails and toenails should be cut short because the tips of fingers and toes will often be used for cavity stimulation.

Basic Cavity-Stimulation Techniques

There are more than two hundred basic qigong massage techniques existing in Chinese history. However, the most common ones number about fifty. Among these fifty, a few of them are specialized in cavity press massage (點穴按摩, dian xue an mo). Here we will introduce a few that serve the purposes of this book.

1. Press and Vibrate with Hand (Zhen Zhan, 震顫). Pressing is used to generate deeper penetration, and the vibration is used for stimulation. The common places of the hand to use to stimulate are the tip of the thumb, index finger, or middle fingers. In order to enhance the pressing and vibrating, usually one or two other fingers is used to support the first joint of the pressing finger. For example, the index finger is used to support the thumb, the thumb is used to support the index finger, or the thumb and the middle finger are used to support the index finger.

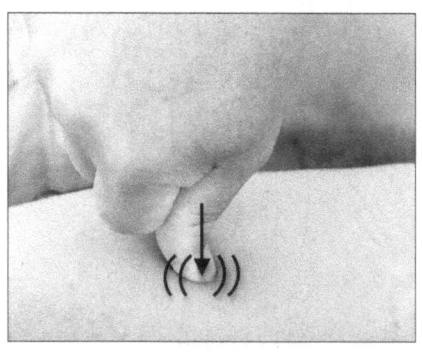
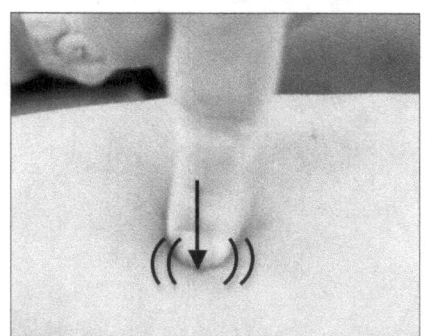

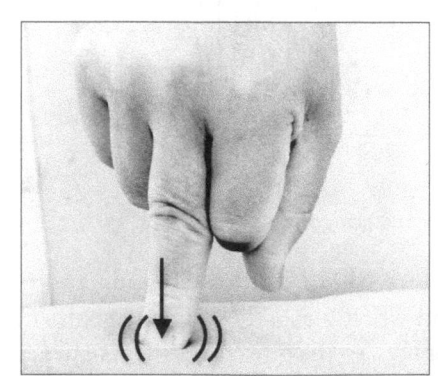

Using the tip of the thumb, index, or middle finger to stimulate.

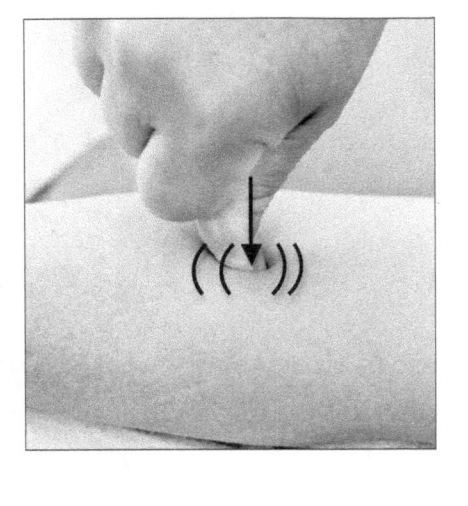

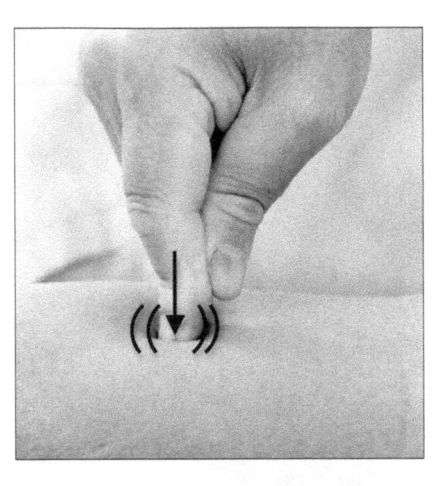

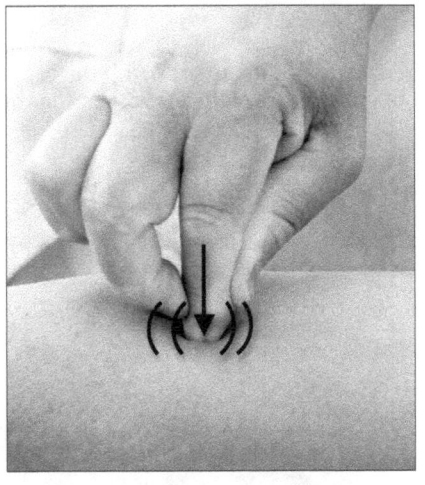

(Pictures from left to right.) Using the index finger to support the thumb, the thumb to support the index finger, and the thumb and middle finger to support the index finger.

Other than fingertips, the knuckles are also commonly used: for example, the knuckle of the thumb with support of the index finger, the second knuckle of the index finger with support of the thumb, the second knuckle of the middle finger with support of all other fingers. Often, the base knuckle of the pinky is also used while holding a fist to stimulate cavities. You can see there are so many options that you can use for cavity stimulation. Even though we demonstrate only a couple of options as examples, you should also try other possibilities. Soon you will realize that some options can be easier and more effective for you than others.

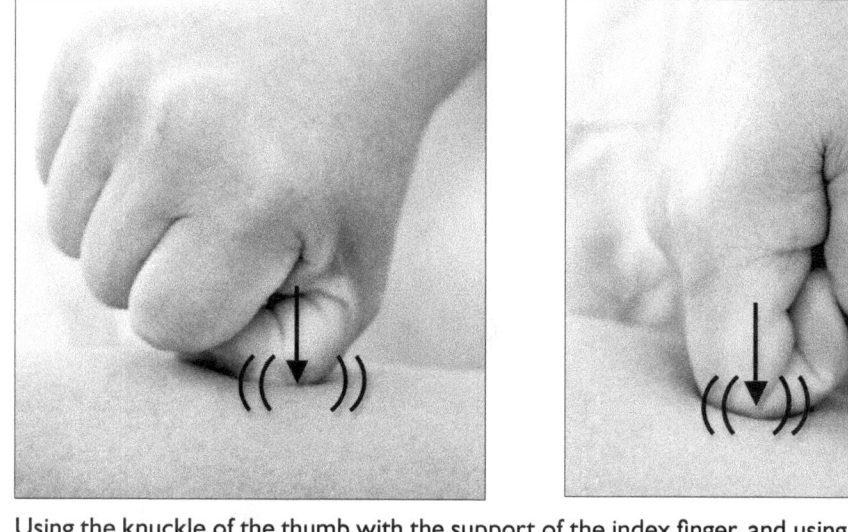

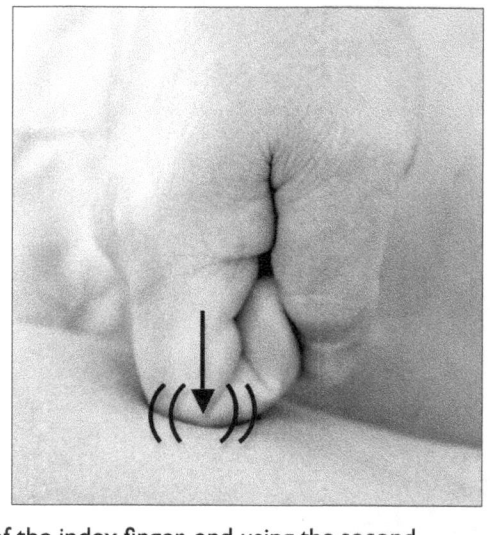

Using the knuckle of the thumb with the support of the index finger, and using the second knuckle of index finger with support of the thumb to stimulate cavities.

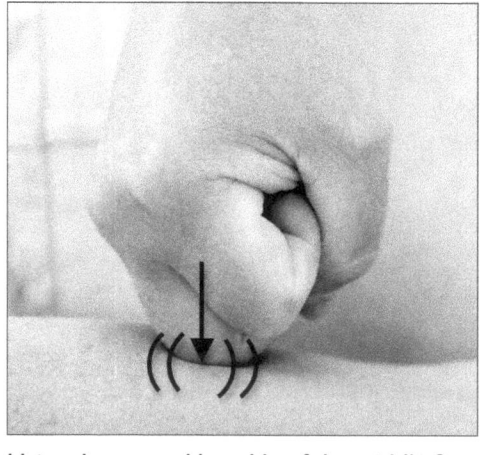

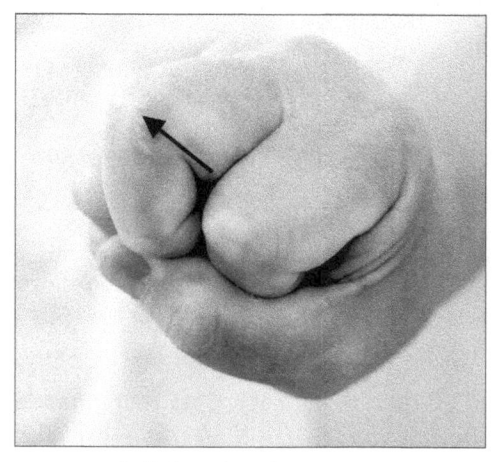

Using the second knuckle of the middle finger with support of all the other fingers.

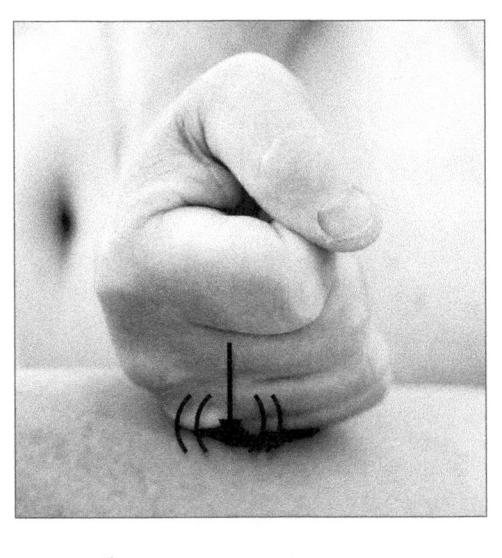

Using the base knuckle of the pinky while holding a fist to stimulate cavities.

2. Press and Vibrate with the Foot (Zhen Zhan, 震顫). Compared to the hand, the foot is much less used for cavity press massage. This is because most people are not skillful in using the foot to massage. However, if you know how to use it, the advantage is that the pressing power can be stronger, but the disadvantage is that the area massaged will be wider than if the hand is used. There are three areas that can be used for cavity press massage. The first is the tip of the big toes. The places massaged usually are the back of the knee or calf. The second area of the foot that can be used for massage is the heel. Usually, the areas covered are the inner side of the leg and foot. Finally, the base knuckle of the small toes can be used to massage the back of your foot.

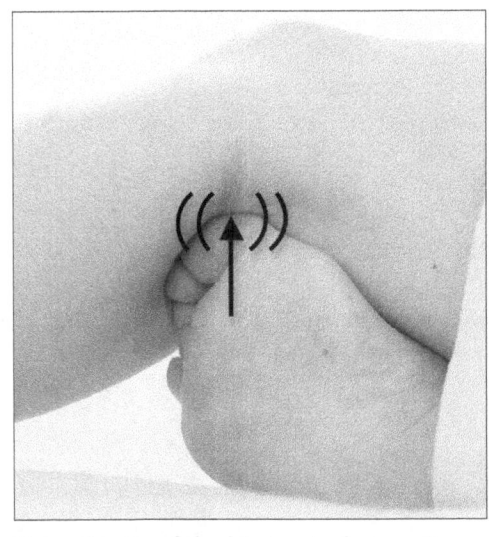

Using the tip of the big toe to do a cavity press on the back of the knee.

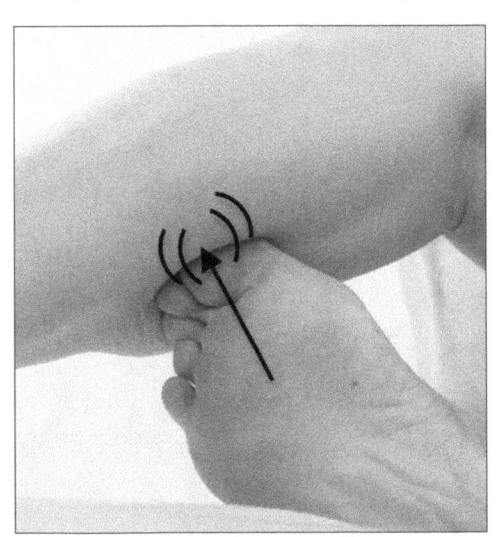

Using the tip of the big toe on the calf.

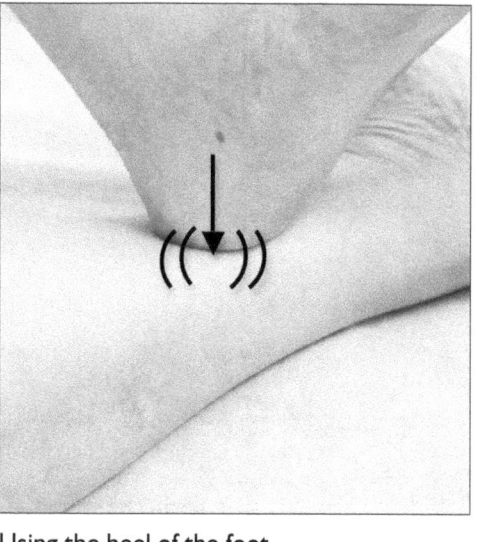

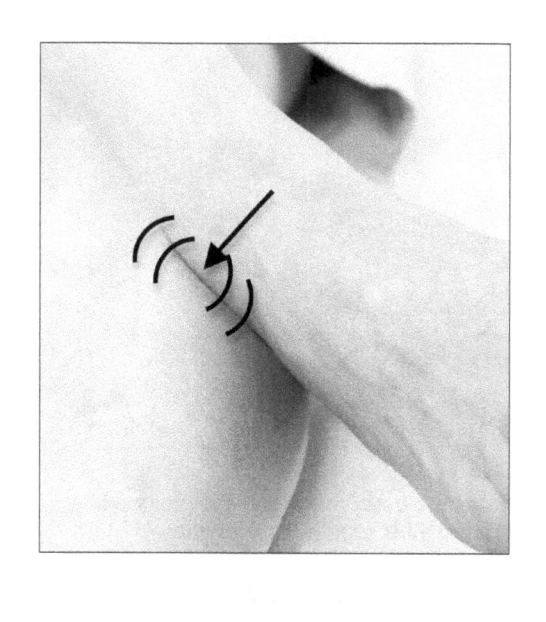

Using the heel of the foot.

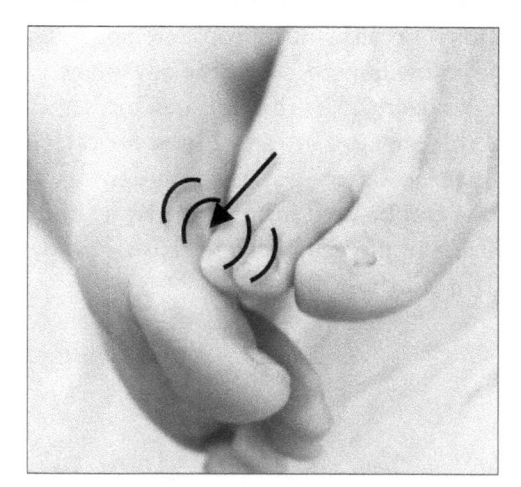

Using the base knuckle of the small toes to massage the back of your foot.

3. Circular Rubbing Motion (Quan Rou, 圈揉). Stabilize your contact, and gently rub with a circular motion. When you use circular rubbing for massage, the power will not be as penetrating as pressing and vibrating. That means you can massage the same areas but reduce the power to half. Often, in order to be more comfortable and cover a bigger area, the front of the thumb, index, or middle finger is used with the support of the other fingers. Frequently, a few fingers can be used together, such as the index and middle fingers or the three middle fingers.

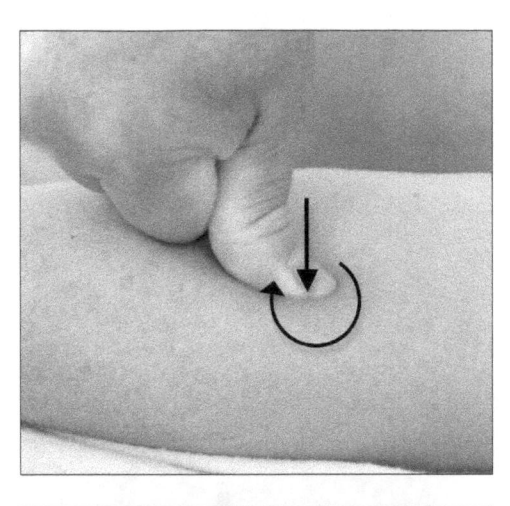

Using the thumb to gently rub with a
circular motion.

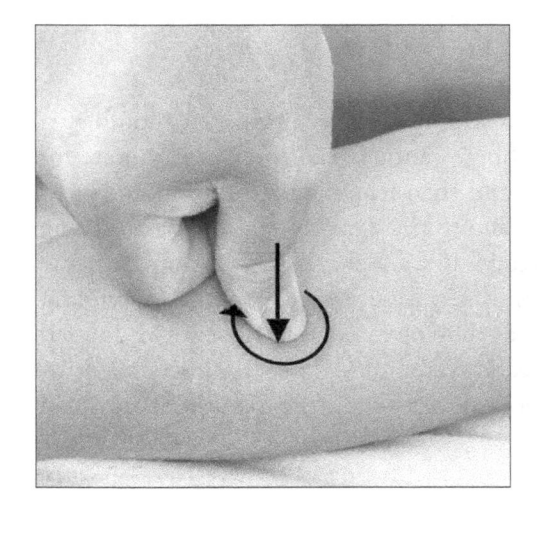

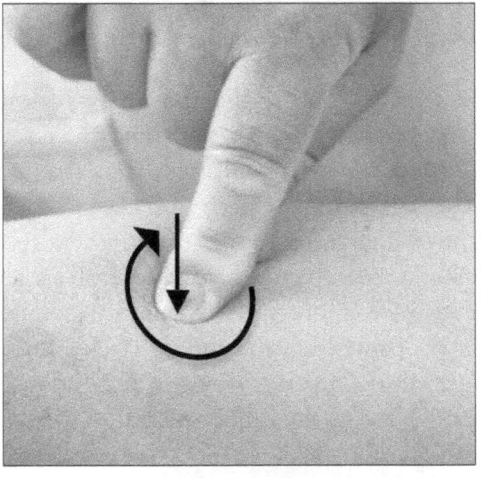

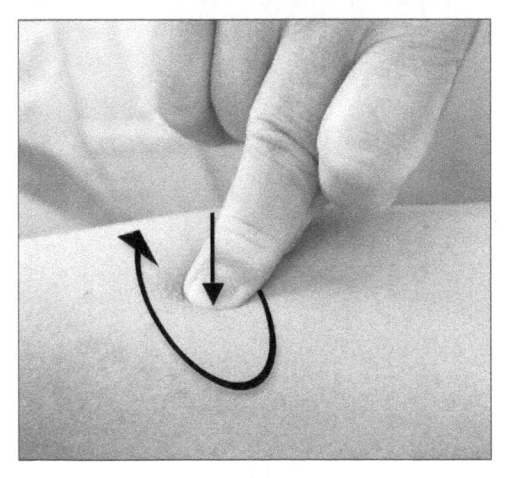

(From left to right.) Using the front of the
thumb. Using the index finger. Using the
middle finger with the support of the other
fingers.

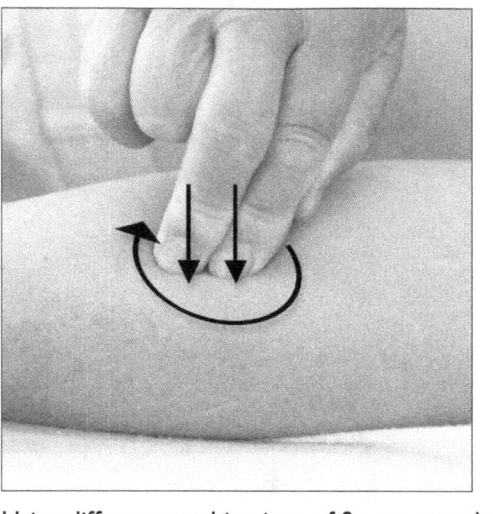 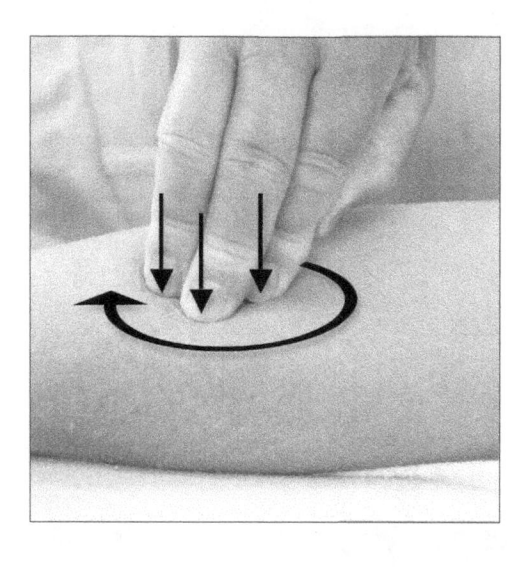

Using different combinations of fingers together.

When you use the above two techniques to stimulate the cavities, you should first use pressing vibration and then the circular rubbing motion. First press and vibrate for ten seconds. After this, rest for a few seconds, and then repeat one or two more times. This will stimulate deep into the cavity area. Then use circular rubbing massage to bring the qi stagnation to the surface and also to spread it to a wider area. When you are using circular rubbing for the cavities, rub for ten seconds, rest for a few seconds, and then repeat one or two more times. When you execute circular rubbing massage, if the cavity is located at the centerline, you should circle in both directions, ten times in each direction. However, if you massage on the side of body, then you want to follow the direction that the qi can be led to the limbs and out.

Massage Sequence

I. Head and Neck (頭、頸部)

1. Top of Head (頭頂)

Begin the massage sequence with the head. Using gentle circles together with press and vibrate will help you to loosen up the fasciae between the skin and skeleton and improve the qi and blood circulation on the top of your head.

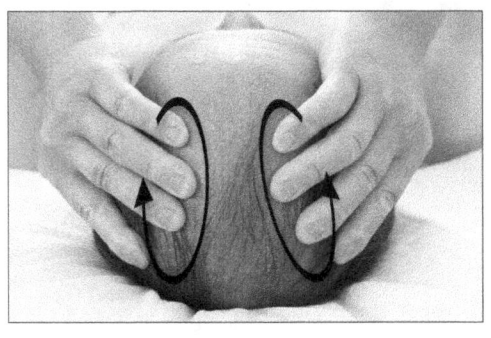

First put both palms on your scalp, and gently circle them.

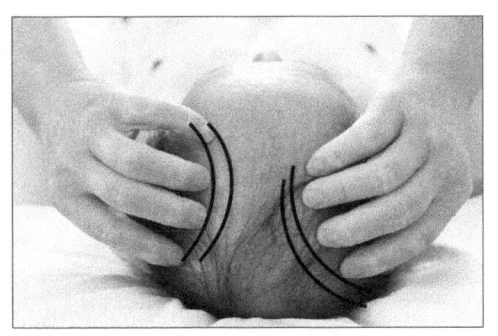

Next use your fingers (avoid fingernails) to press the skin of your head, and vibrate them gently. Begin from the center, and then move to the sides—from the forehead, then gradually to the back.

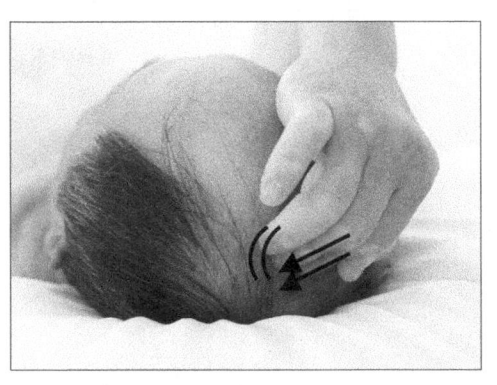

Next use your index and middle fingers to press, and gently vibrate the baihui cavity at the top of your head (百會, GV-20) for ten seconds. Then gently rub the area in a circular motion ten times in each direction.

Massaging baihui can help ailments such as headache, lightheadedness, hemorrhoids, wind stroke, seizures, insanity, extreme nervousness, shock, high blood pressure, deafness, tinnitus, low blood pressure, a hangover, dizziness, fainting, coma, insomnia, irritability, chronic diarrhea, and so forth. Circle in each direction twenty to thirty times.

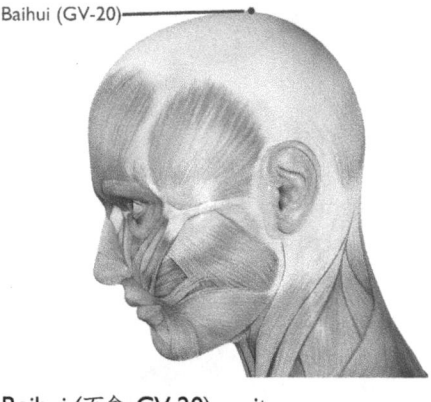

Baihui (GV-20)

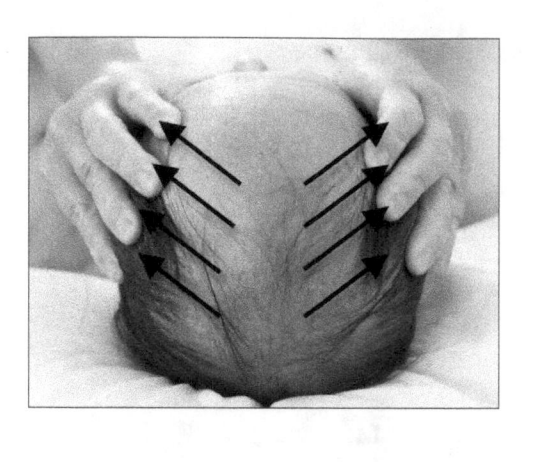

Baihui (百會, GV-20) cavity.

Finally, use all five fingers to press and push from the center of the head to the sides (ten times).

2. Center of Face (面中)

Massaging the face is an important part of Chinese medicine.

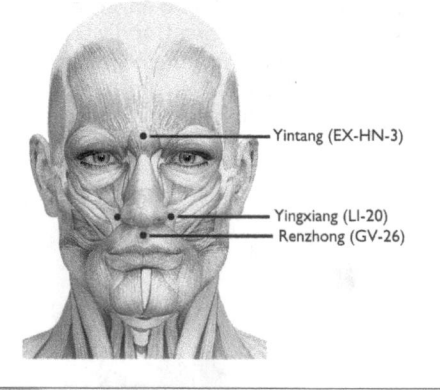

Yintang (EX-HN-3)

Yingxiang (LI-20)
Renzhong (GV-26)

Yintang (印堂, EX-HN-3), yingxiang (迎香, LI-20), and renzhong (人中, GV-26) cavities.

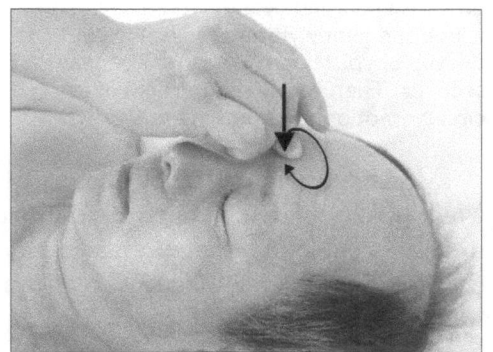

Use your middle finger to press and vibrate the yintang cavity, your third eye area (印堂, EX-HN-3) for ten seconds. Repeat. Then gently circle the cavity ten times in each direction.

Massaging the yintang cavity/third eye can relieve conditions such as headache, rhinitis, swollen red eyes, trigeminal neuralgia, insomnia, hypertension, nasal congestion, runny nose, dizziness, and eye disease.

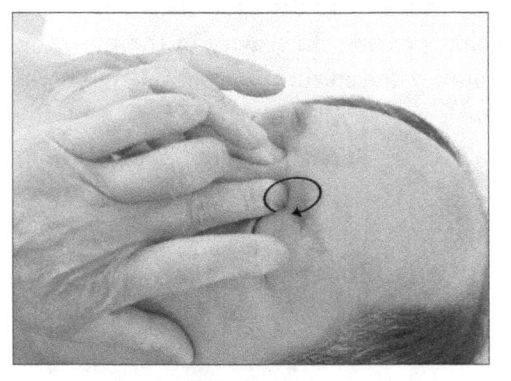

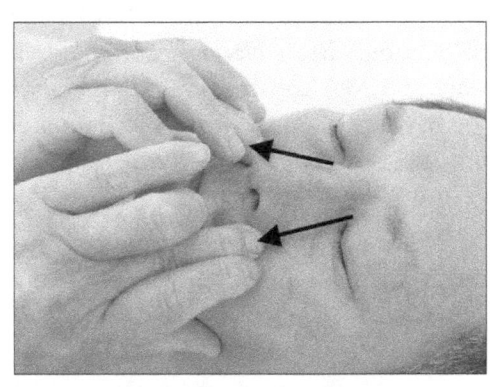

Next use the middle fingers to gently massage the upper area of the nose, between the eyes. Gently rub the area in a circular motion five times. This will release sinus pressure.

Next use the middle fingers to push downward along the sides of the nose until they reach the yingxiang (迎香, LI-20) cavities. Use your index or middle finger tip to press and vibrate these two cavities with good pressure for ten seconds. Repeat one more time. Then rub the area with a circular motion ten times in each direction.

Stimulating yingxiang cavities can alleviate symptoms of nasal obstruction, nose disorders, smelling problems, nasal polyp, flu, wind-heat and wind-cold, facial paralysis, and facial skin problems. These points are also known for having antiaging effects, such as improving circulation to improve the wrinkling and sagging skin of the face.

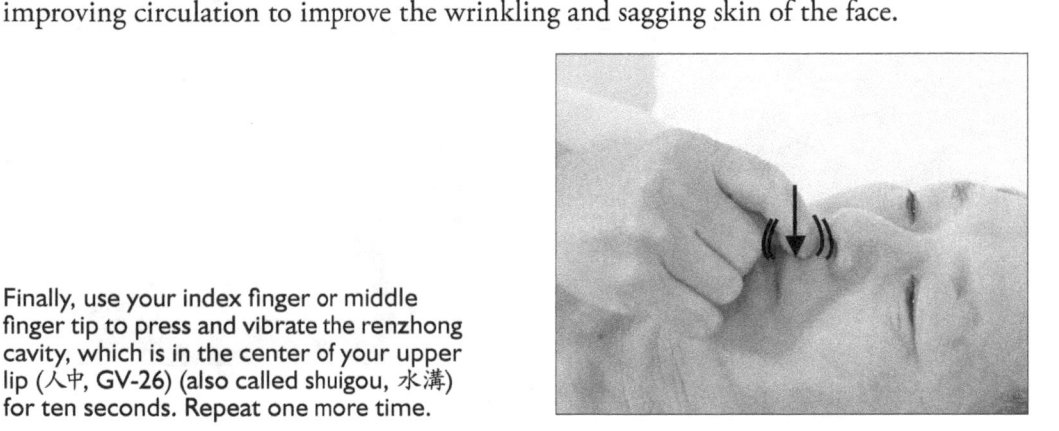

Finally, use your index finger or middle finger tip to press and vibrate the renzhong cavity, which is in the center of your upper lip (人中, GV-26) (also called shuigou, 水溝) for ten seconds. Repeat one more time.

Renzhong cavity is the main point for restoring consciousness after shock, fainting, and weakness; it also helps with wind stroke, collapse syndrome, seizures, hysteria, lock-jaw, facial paralysis or swelling, eye twitches, spine pain and muscle spasms, acute lower back pain and stiffness, nasal blockage, rhinitis, summer heat diseases, chest pain, and palpitations. Moreover, it is commonly known that pressing this cavity in the morning wakes up your conscious mind and raises your vitality and spirit.

Repeat the entire process for two more times.

3. Sides of Face (面側)

Begin this massage by using your middle fingers to circulate the sinus area between the eyes, as you did at the start of the previous massage. Circle five times.

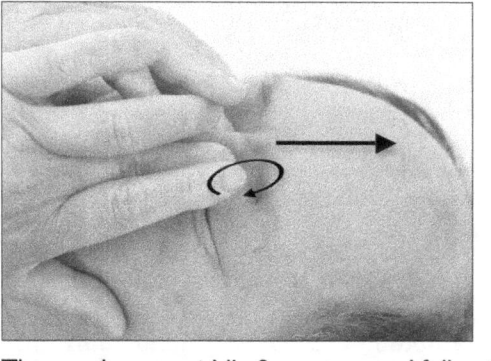
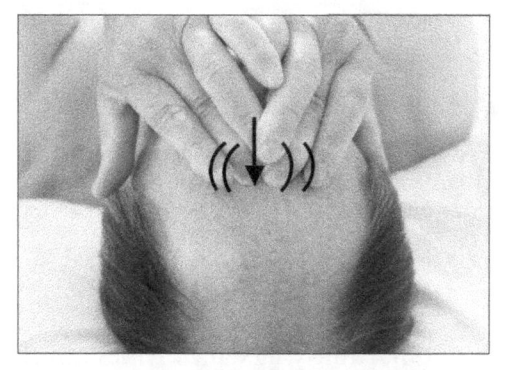

Then push your middle fingers upward following the centerline of your forehead until they reach the shenting (神庭, GV-24) cavity. Use your middle finger to press and vibrate the cavity for ten seconds. Repeat one more time.

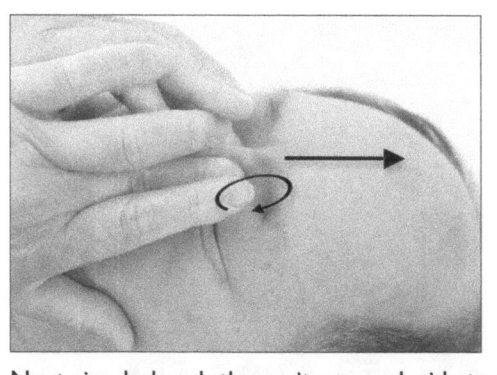
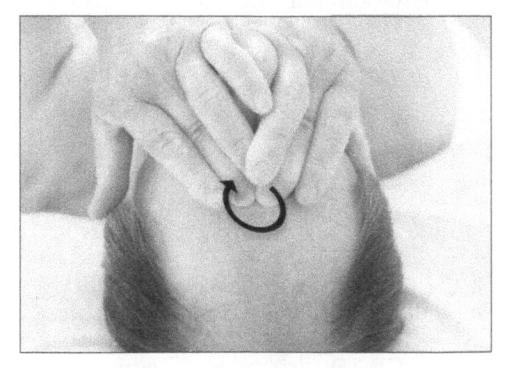

Next circularly rub the cavity on each side ten times.

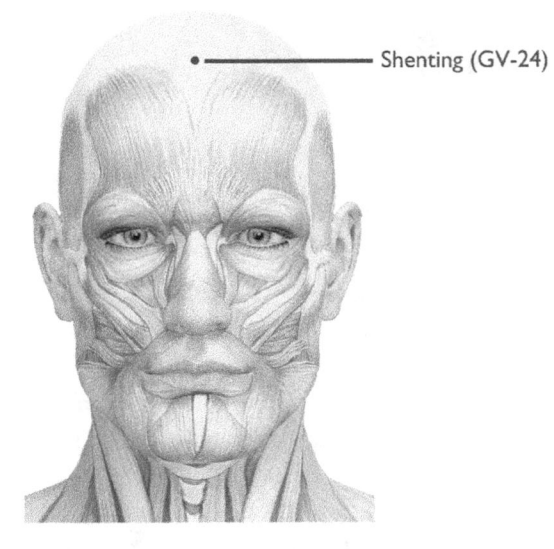

Shenting (神庭, **GV-24**) cavity.

Shenting (神庭, GV-24) cavity is known for treating epilepsy, palpitation, insomnia, frontal headache, dizziness, and chronic sinusitis, nosebleeds, nasal discharge, vomiting, and excessive tearing. Psychologically, this cavity can treat anxiety, panic attacks, fear, incoordination, mad behavior, and bi-polar disorder. Massaging this cavity in the morning is useful to help you find the spiritual center.

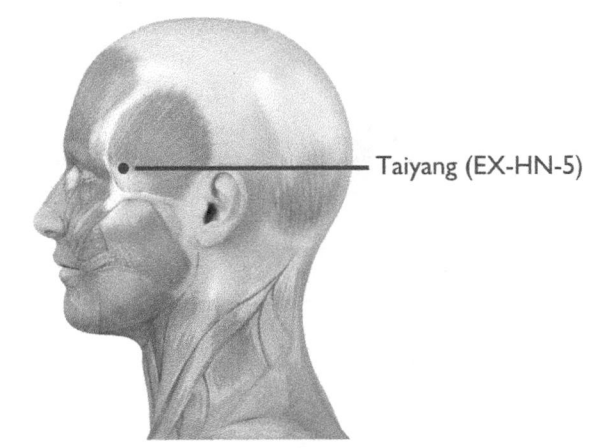

Taiyang (太陽) (**EX-HN-5**) (left and right temples).

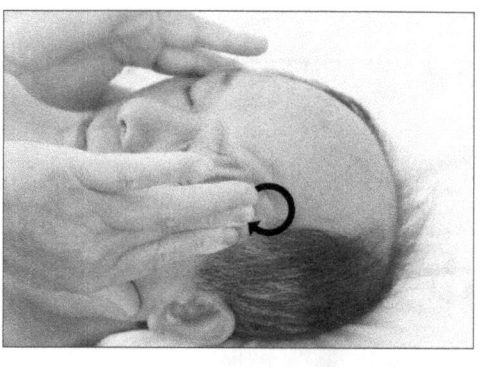

Using your index and middle fingers, gently rub the temples in a circular motion moving up, back, down, and around. This direction is used for releasing the pressure. Circle the cavities for ten seconds. This will help you to release the head's tension and relax. Repeat one more time.

Next use your index and middle fingers to push along the edge of the hairline to the sides and then down to taiyang (太陽) (left and right temples) (EX-HN-5).

If you reverse the direction, you are leading the qi upward, and the energy can be trapped on your head, which can consequently make your headache or head tension worse. Normally, the circular rubbing motion can effectively serve the purpose. If you like to add press with vibration, you must be very gentle.

Taiyang (太陽) (left and right temples) (EX-HN-5) are the most common cavities for massage when you have headache, eye disorders, and facial paralysis. It has also been commonly recognized that by massaging these two cavities, you are able to relieve fatigue, raise the spirit of vitality, and prevent hair loss.

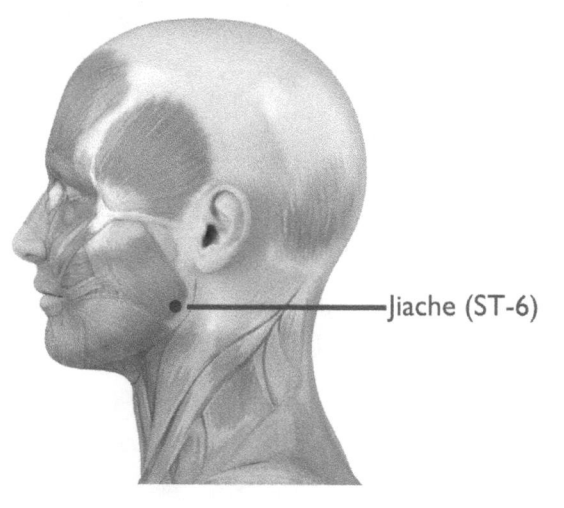

Jiache (ST-6)

Jiache (頰車) (ST-6) cavity.

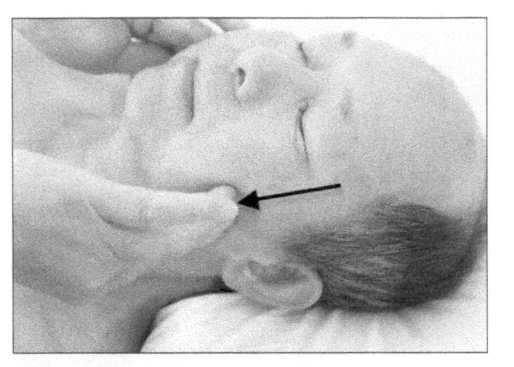 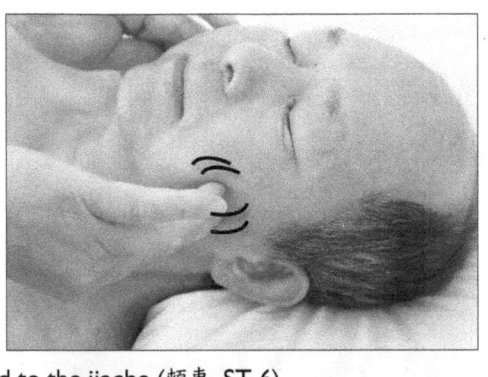

Next push your index and middle fingers downward to the jiache (頰車, ST-6) (牙腮) cavities on both sides of the lower jaw, below the cheeks. Use your index and middle fingers to press and vibrate the cavities for ten seconds. Repeat one more time.

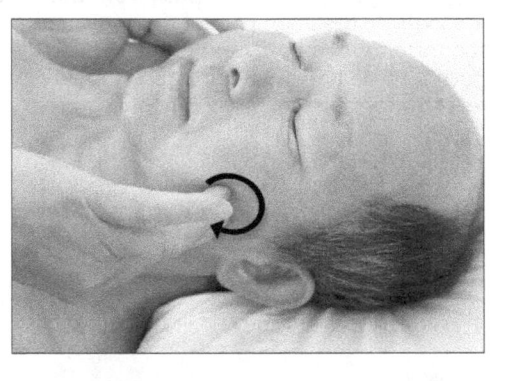

Then rub the cavity area in a circular motion. Circle upward, backward, down, and around.

Jiache (頰車, ST-6) cavities are commonly used to treat facial paralysis, neck pain and stiffness, sore throat, toothache, edema of the face, mumps, and lockjaw. Massaging these cavities on both sides of the lower jaw, below the cheeks, can also stimulate the function of the glands producing saliva.

Repeat the entire process two more times.

4. Eyes (眼)

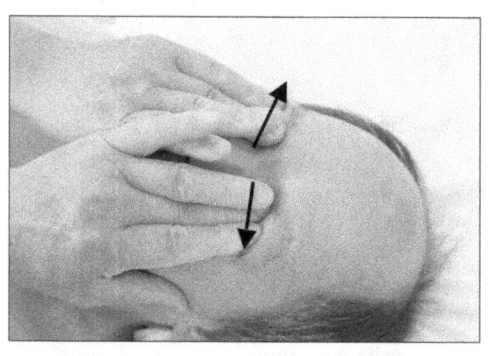

Use the tips of your index and middle fingers to gently press and push from the area where the inner part of the eyes meets the nose to the outer sides of the eyes. Push it three times. The pressure should feel comfortable.

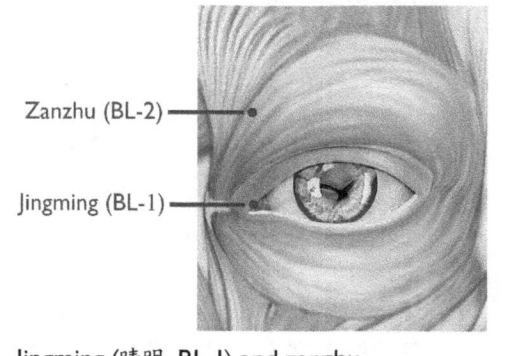

Zanzhu (BL-2)

Jingming (BL-1)

Jingming (晴明, BL-1) and zanzhu (攢竹, BL-2) cavities.

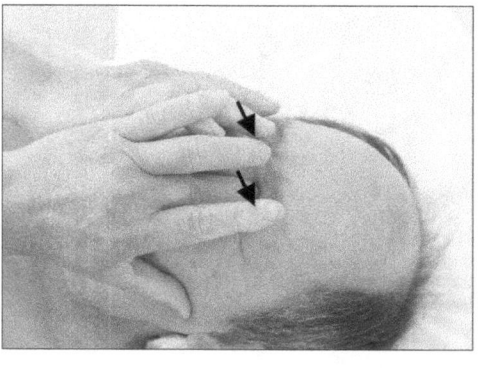

Then use the tip of the index finger to gently but firmly press and vibrate the jingming (晴明, BL-1) cavity. This cavity is located where the inner part of the eye meets the nose, also known as the inner canthus. Gently stimulate it for five seconds, and then relax. Repeat two more times.

Massaging the jingming (晴明, BL-1) cavity is used to treat all kinds of eye conditions: conjunctivitis, myopia, glaucoma, blurred vision, optic nerve atrophy, night and color blindness, excessive tearing, itching, cataract, retinitis, dizziness, and pituitary and pineal gland diseases.

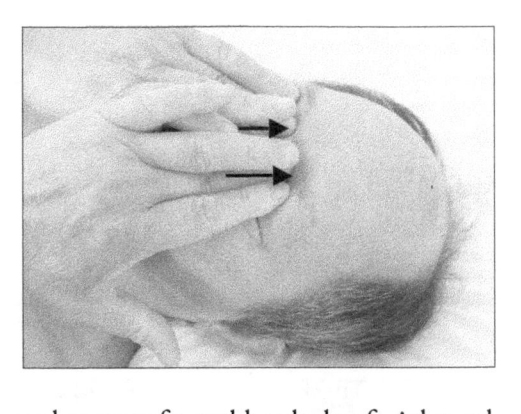

Next move your index finger up to the eyebrow area and press the zanzhu (攢竹, BL-2) cavity. This cavity lies in the depression at the inner ends of the eyebrows. Again, gently stimulate it for five seconds, and then relax. Repeat two more times.

Zanzhu (攢竹, BL-2) cavity is commonly used to treat frontal headache, facial paralysis, blurred vision, weak eyesight, eye diseases in general, glaucoma, tearing, dizziness, conjunctivitis, sinusitis, rhinitis, allergies affecting the eyes and nose, itching, sneezing, red and painful eyes, myopia, cataract, and acute lower back pain or sprain.

These two cavities often work together and are perhaps the best two points for all kinds of eye problems from early-stage cataracts or glaucoma to hysteria with vision loss. They are also used for problems with conjunctivitis due to wind-heat and liver-heat, and for blurred vision in the elderly due to deficient jing (精, essence) and xue (血, blood).

After finishing the stimulation of these two cavities, repeat the pushing motion from the inner edge of eyes to the outer sides of the eyes three times. Repeat the entire process one more time.

5. Front and Behind Ears (耳前、耳後)

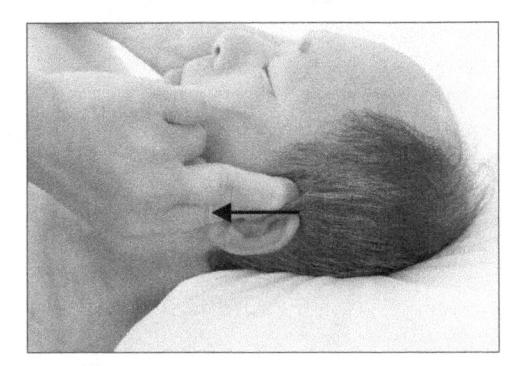

Next use your index and middle fingers to push along the line right in front of the ear from top to the bottom. Repeat nine times.

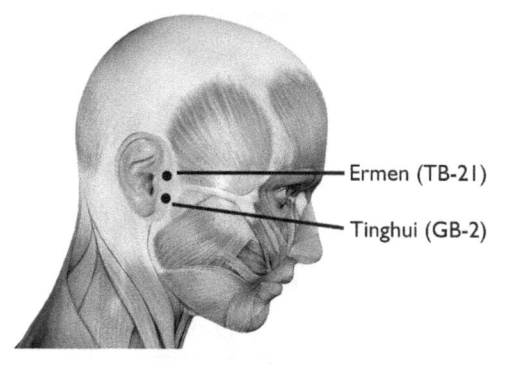

Ermen (耳門, TB-21) and tinghui (聽會, GB-2) cavities.

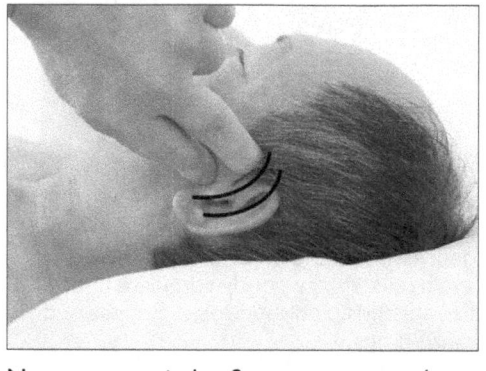

Next use your index finger to press and vibrate the ermen (耳門, TB-21) cavity for ten seconds. Repeat two more times.

Stimulating the ermen cavity can treat tinnitus, deafness, impaired hearing, earache, discharge of pus from the ear, toothache, headache, swelling of the ear, and ear sores.

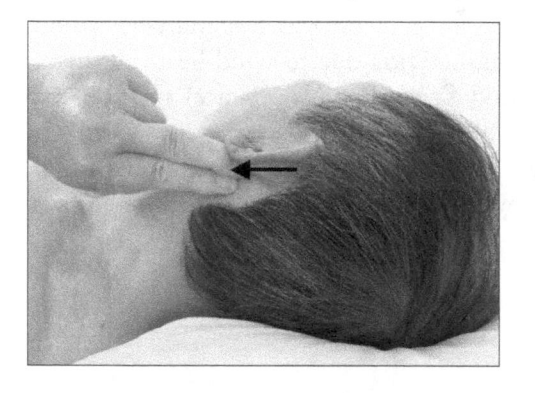

Then move your index finger down to the tinghui (聽會, GB-2) cavity and repeat the same process. Stimulate it for ten seconds, and repeat two times.

Massaging the tinghui cavity can benefit the ears, eliminate wind, and relieve headache, toothache, mumps, seizures, sadness, deafness, tinnitus, joint arthritis of the jaw (TMJ), convulsions, and facial paralysis or pain. It can also clear heat, and activate the channels and alleviate pain.

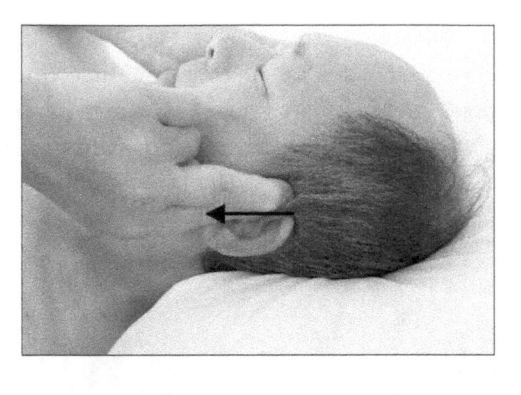

Follow the front line of the ear from top to the bottom for ten times.

If you like, you may repeat the entire process one more time.

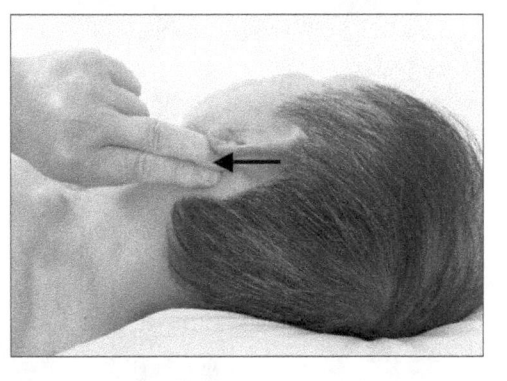

Next use your index and middle fingers to push and rub downward on the back of the ear from top to bottom. Repeat nine times.

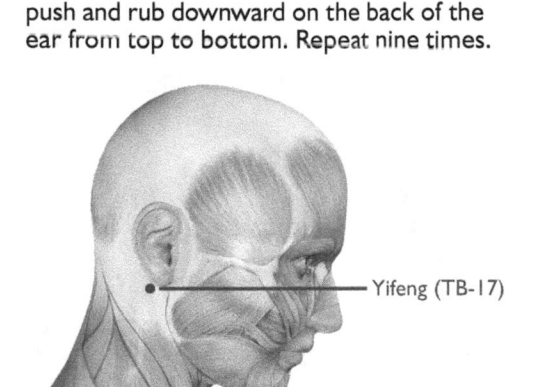

Yifeng (翳風, TB-17) cavity.

Then use your index finger to gently push and stimulate the yifeng (翳風, TB-17) cavity. Stimulate it for ten seconds. Repeat two times. After you finish stimulation of this cavity, repeat the pushing action used at the beginning of this front-and-behind massage sequence of the ears.

Massaging the yifeng (翳風, TB-17) cavity will expel (external) wind, benefit the ears, clear heat, open the channel and luo-connecting vessels (絡, luo) (i.e., secondary qi channels), and alleviate pain. Therefore, it can be used to treat facial paralysis, lockjaw, trigeminal neuralgia, convulsions, tinnitus, deafness, otitis media, blurred vision, vertigo, aural hallucinations, toothache, swelling of the cheek, and scrofula.

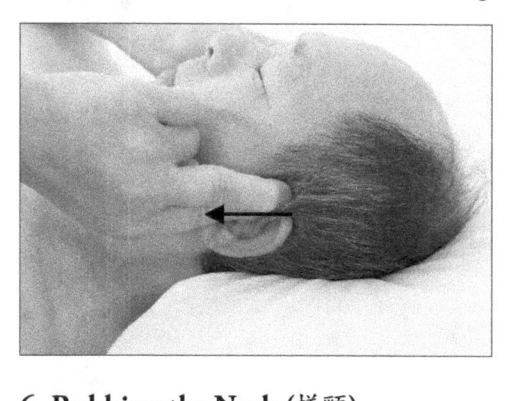

After you finish stimulation of this cavity, repeat the pushing action following the front line of the ear from top to bottom ten times. If you like, you may repeat the entire process one more time.

6. Rubbing the Neck (搓頸)

Be very gentle when rubbing the neck.

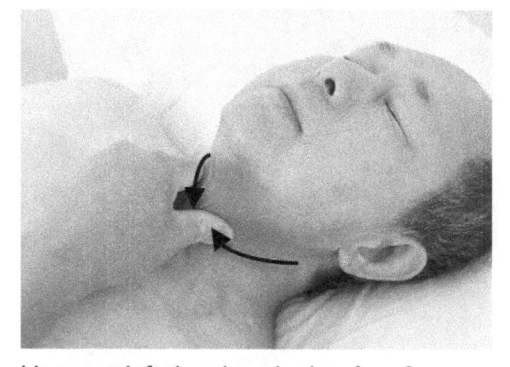

Use your left thumb and other four fingers to rub the front of your neck gently from the sides to the front centerline ten times. Then change hands, and repeat the same rubbing motions ten times. Remember, your rubbing should be very gentle and make you feel comfortable.

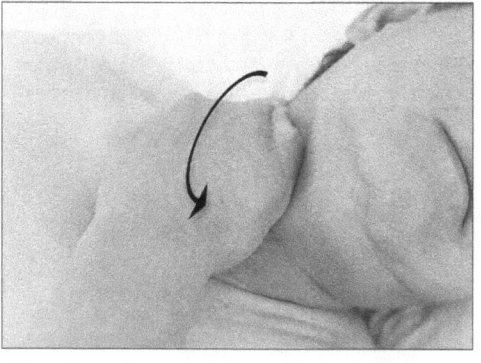

After this, use your left hand to rub the right side of the back of your neck, from the back to the side ten times. Repeat the same process for the other side by using your right hand.

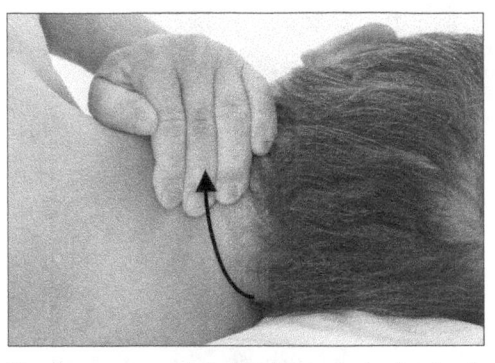

Finally, use your left hand to rub the back of the neck from the right to the left ten times. Do not lift up your head because it will cause tension and prevent you from reaching the deeper area of the back of the neck. Repeat the same process from the other side using the right hand.

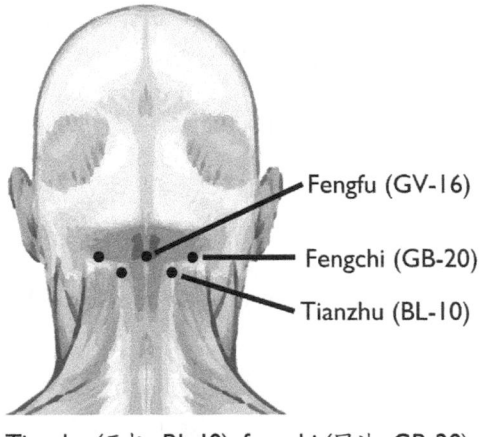

Fengfu (GV-16)

Fengchi (GB-20)

Tianzhu (BL-10)

Tianzhu (天柱, BL-10), fengchi (風池, GB-20), and fengfu (風府, GV-16) cavities.

Now use your right index and middle fingers to stimulate the following three cavities: tianzhu (天柱, BL-10), fengchi (風池, GB-20), and fengfu (風府, GV-16).

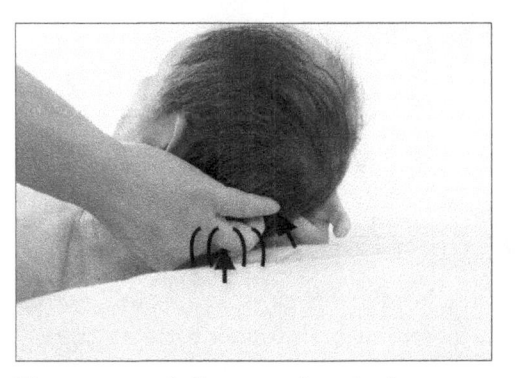

First press and vibrate each cavity for ten seconds. Repeat one more time.

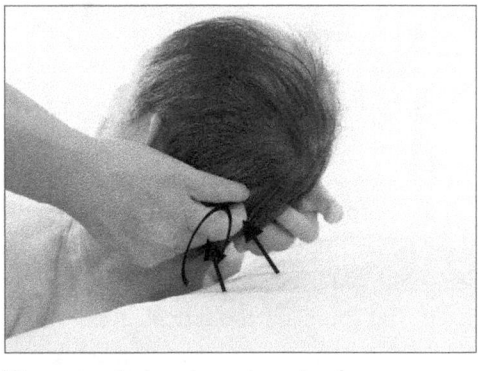

Then circularly rub each cavity for ten seconds, circling from the central line upward, outward, and back around.

Massaging the tianzhu (天柱, BL-10) cavity will relieve occipital headache, neck pain and stiffness, lower back pain, dizziness, convulsions in children, epilepsy, eye diseases, laryngitis, nasal obstruction, heaviness of the head, swollen throat, weak limbs and lack of coordination, and neurasthenia.

Massaging the fengchi (風池, GB-20) cavity can help febrile diseases, headache, migraine, common cold and flu, hypertension, cerebral hemorrhage and congestion, glaucoma, dizziness, insomnia, stiffness of the neck and nape, blurred vision, optic nerve atrophy, conjunctivitis, tinnitus, vertigo, aural vertigo, convulsion, infantile convulsion, seizures, fever, common cold, flushed face, stuffy nose, and skin diseases.

Stimulating the fengfu (風府, GV-16) cavity is used to treat headache, dizziness, neck rigidity, blurred vision, flu, wind rash, rhinitis, sinusitis, blocked nose, vertigo, cerebral hemorrhage, seizures, fear, anxiety, suicidal behavior, sore throat, postapoplectic aphasia, and ceaseless vomiting.

7. Massage the Jianjing (肩井, GB-21) (肩井按摩)

The last step of massaging the head and neck is to lead the qi away. The major cavity to serve this purpose is the jianjing (肩井, GB-21).

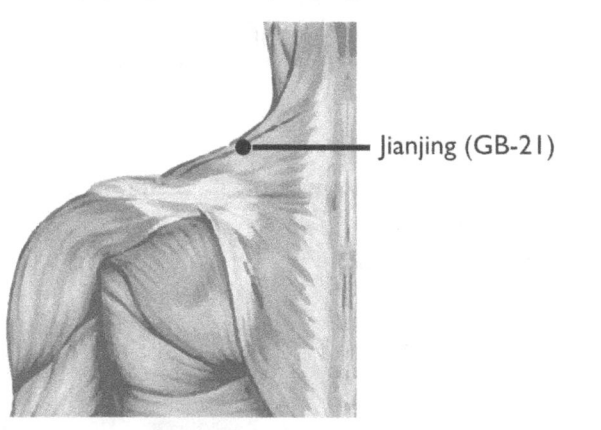

Jianjing (GB-21)

Jianjing (肩井, GB-21) cavity.

The jianjing cavity is located by first pinching the shoulder muscle between your thumb and middle finger. It is well known that massaging the tendons between the neck and shoulders, and also the jianjing cavity, eases tension of the head and neck. It is also well recognized that these are the crucial areas and cavities to loosening up the upper back and arms.

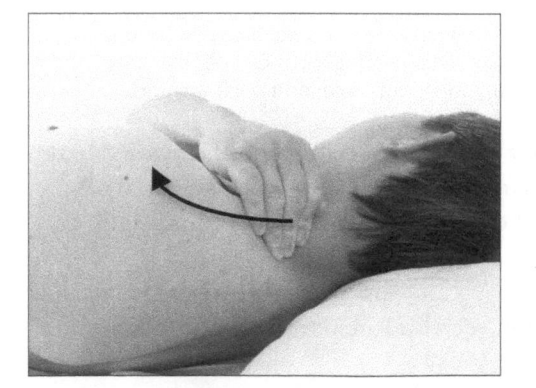

First use your right-hand fingers to push the tendon connecting the neck and left shoulder. Push from the neck to the left shoulder ten times.

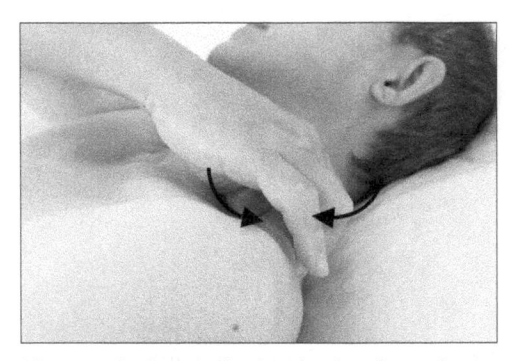

Next grab the tendon and rub it from the neck area to the left shoulder. Repeat 2 more times.

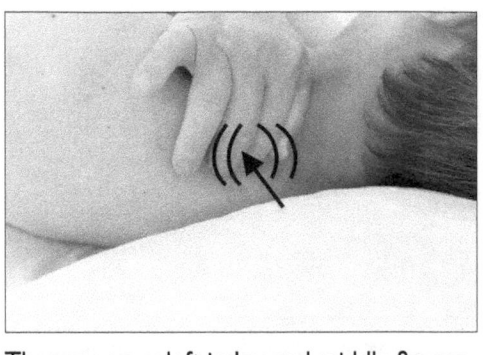

Then use your left index and middle fingers to press and vibrate the jianjing cavity for ten seconds. Repeat one more time. Finally, use your right-hand fingers to again push the tendon from the neck to the left shoulder ten times.

After you have completed massaging the left side using your right hand, repeat the same process for the right side using your left hand.

The jianjing (肩井, GB-21) cavity is most commonly used for stiffness and pain of the neck, tension of the shoulders and upper back, mastitis, difficult labor, scrofula, vertigo, headaches, chest pain, boils, carbuncles, breast abscess, alternate hot and cold, fever, blurred vision, optic nerve atrophy, tinnitus, poor hearing, stiffness of the spine, and nausea.

8. Massage the Jianyu (肩髃, LI-15) (肩髃按摩)

Now, continue to stimulate the jianyu cavity located at the shoulder joints. There are two purposes for stimulating this cavity. First you will lead the qi away from the head and neck continuously. Next you will stimulate and excite the area of the shoulder joints, so this junction between the torso and arm can be loosened and opened.

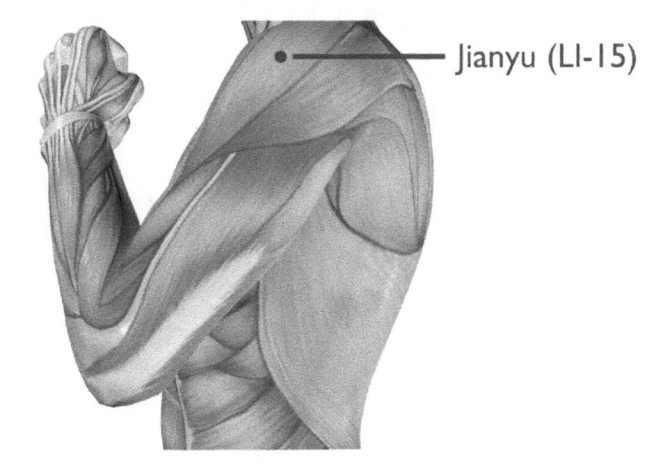

Jianyu (LI-15)

Jianyu (肩髃, LI-15) cavity.

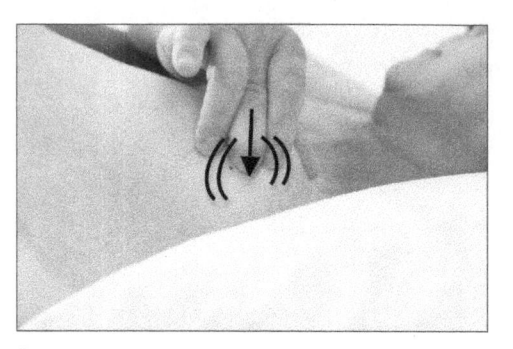

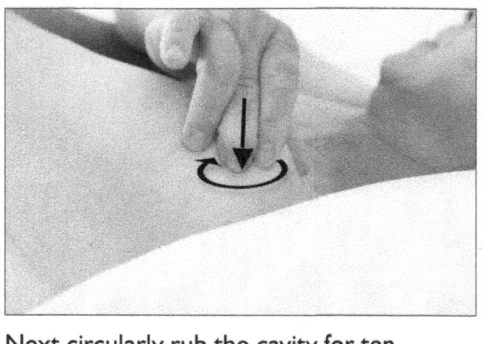

First use your right index or middle finger to firmly press and vibrate the jianyu (肩髃, LI-15) cavity on the left shoulder for ten seconds. Relax for a few seconds, and then repeat for another ten seconds.

Next circularly rub the cavity for ten seconds, and repeat one more time. Naturally, after you finish massaging one side, you treat the other side.

The jianyu cavity is known for treating all kinds of shoulder disorders, rotator cuff injuries, adhesive capsulitis, frozen shoulder, paralysis of the arm, scrofula, afflictions of shoulder joint and muscles, hemiplegia, excessive perspiration, goiter, dry skin, and spermatorrhea.

9. Massage the Jianneiling (肩內陵, M-UE-48) (肩內陵按摩)

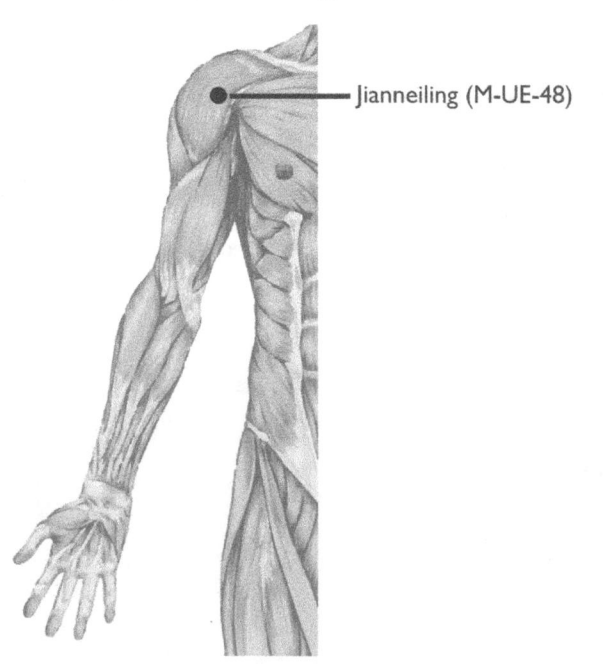

Jianneiling (肩內陵, M-UE-48) cavity.

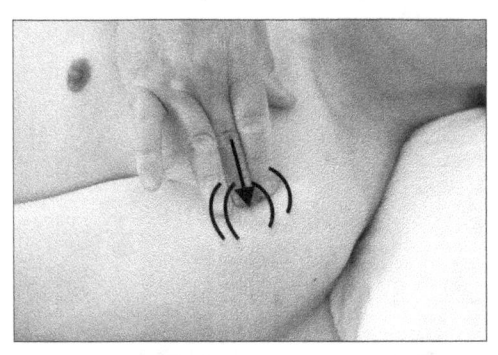

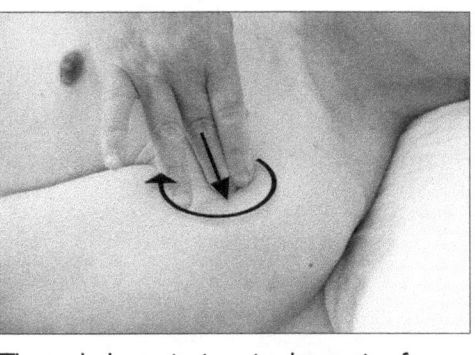

Use your middle finger to press and vibrate the jianneiling (肩內陵, M-UE-48) cavity for ten seconds. Rest for a few seconds, and repeat one more time.

Then rub the cavity in a circular motion for another ten seconds. Repeat one more time.

Stimulating the jianneiling cavity can treat hemiplegia, hypertension, pain in the shoulder joint, inflammation of the shoulder joint, numbness, paralysis and immobility of the shoulder joint, excessive sweating, wind-dampness in the shoulder, arm weakness, goiter, stiffness and pain of the anterior aspect of the shoulder, and frozen shoulder.

II. Front Torso (胸、腹部)

1. Sides of the Upper Chest (上胸側部)

After you have finished the head and neck massage, move down to the front torso area.

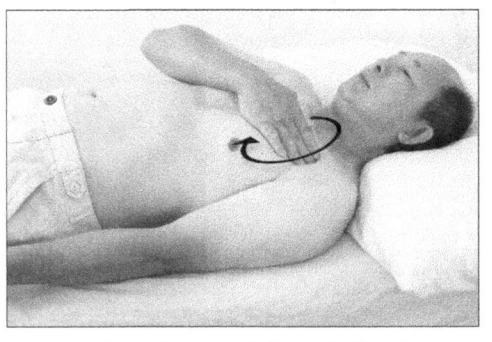

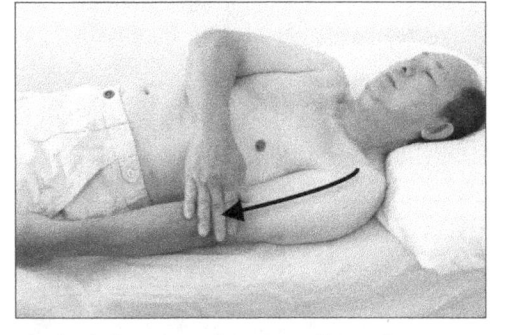

First use four fingers of the right hand to circularly rub the left upper chest area from the cavity area upward, outward, and back around, and then push to the left upper arm. Repeat nine more times.

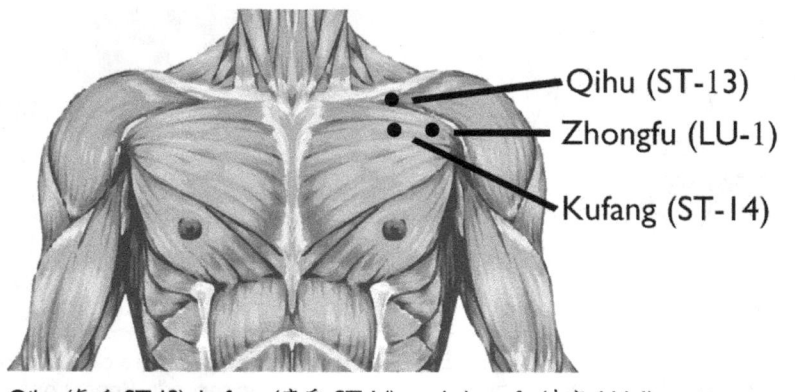

Qihu (氣戶, ST-13), kufang (庫房, ST-14), and zhongfu (中府, LU-1) cavities.

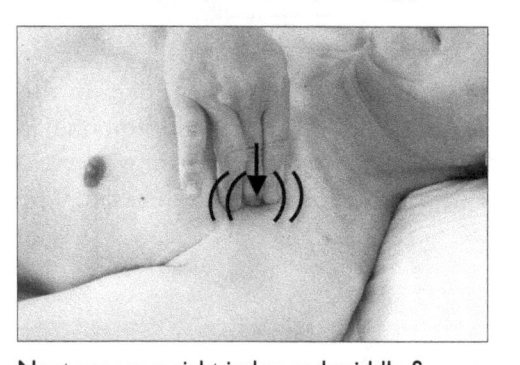

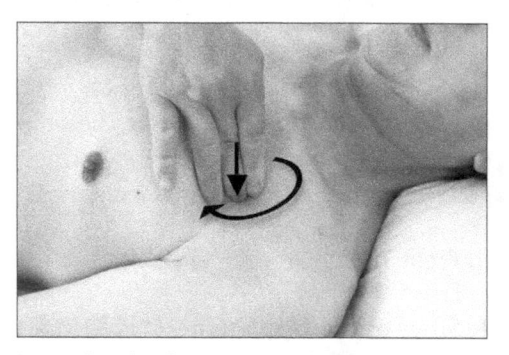

Next use your right index and middle fingers to press and vibrate the qihu (氣戶, ST-13) cavity on your left side for ten seconds. Rest for a few seconds, and repeat for another ten seconds.

Immediately after press and vibrate, rub the cavity in a circular motion, moving from the cavity upward, outward, and back around for ten seconds. Rest for a few seconds, and repeat for another ten seconds.

Next repeat the same stimulating process for the next two cavities: the kufang (庫房, ST-14) and the zhongfu (中府, LU-1).

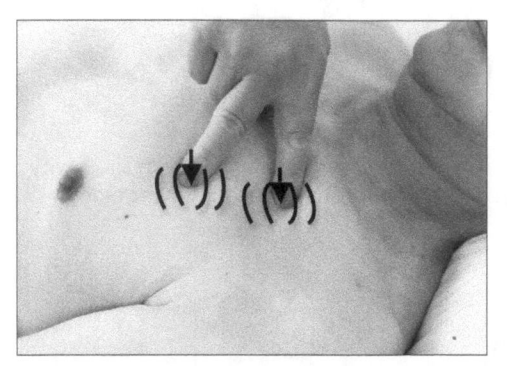

If you prefer, you may use your index and middle fingers to stimulate any two cavities at the same time.

After you finish the stimulation of these three cavities, repeat the same rubbing massage as in the beginning by using the right four fingers to circularly rub the left upper chest area from the cavity area upward, outward, and back around. Next change to the other side, and repeat the entire process.

Qihu means "qi door" in Chinese because it is the boundary of the lungs and surrounding tissues. Qihu (氣戶, ST-13) is commonly used for treating problems such as heaviness of the chest, dyspnea, pleurisy, bronchitis, cough, diaphragm spasm, loss of taste and smell, loss of appetite, and feet perspiration.

The kufang (庫房, ST-14) cavity is used to treat distending pain in the chest and coughing. Zhongfu (中府, LU-1) can be used for treating chest fullness; pneumonia; lung abscess; asthma; bronchitis; wheezing; dyspnea; edema; throat obstruction; chest fullness and pain; neck, back, and shoulder pain; excessive perspiration; dry cough; stuttering; and bad-smelling urine.

2. Central Chest (胸中部)

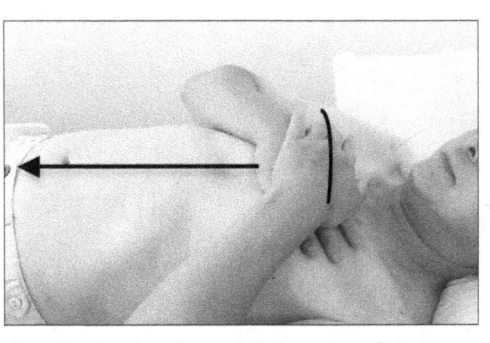

Overlap both palms at the center of the upper chest area. Push and slide your hands downward from the upper chest to the abdominal area ten times.

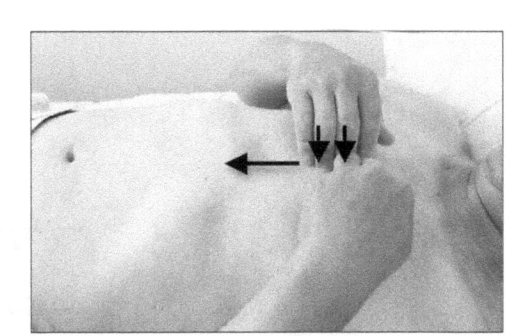

Next use your fingertips to gently tap the centerline from the upper chest to the sternum. Repeat nine times.

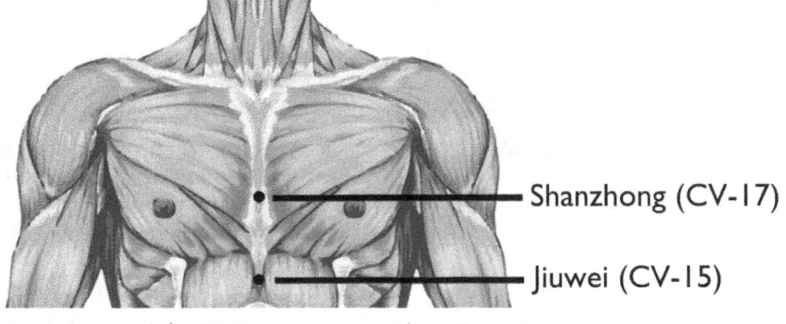

Shanzhong (膻中, CV-17) and jiuwei (鳩尾, CV-15) cavities.

Shanzhong (CV-17)

Jiuwei (CV-15)

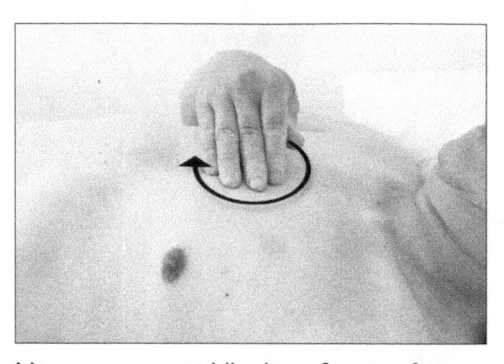

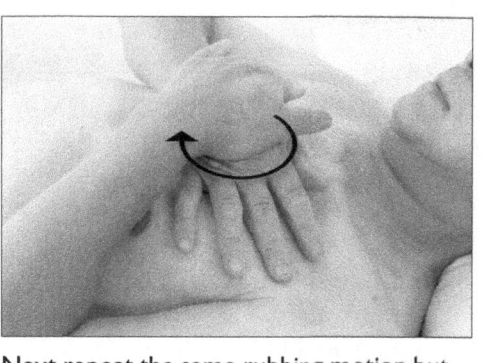

Next use your middle three fingers of your right hand to rub the shanzhong (膻中, CV-17) cavity with a circular motion ten times. Use the other hand to rub the same cavity in the opposite direction ten more times.

Next repeat the same rubbing motion but using your palm instead of fingers ten times in each direction.

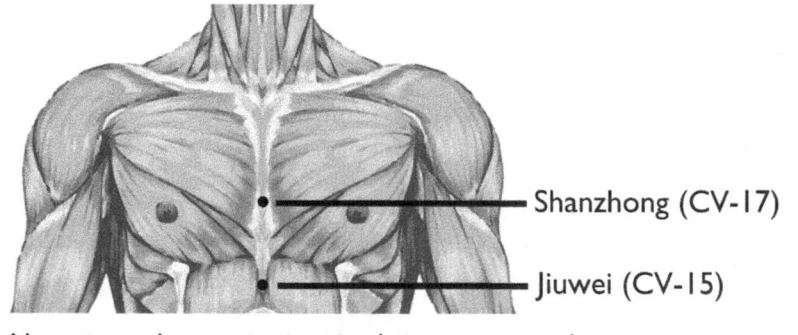

Shanzhong (CV-17)

Jiuwei (CV-15)

Next repeat the same cavity stimulating process to the jiuwei (鳩尾, CV-15) cavity.

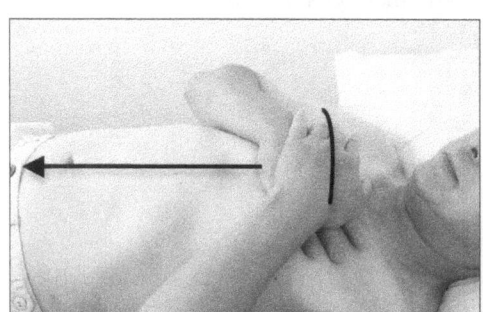

After you have completed the stimulation of these two cavities, repeat the same push and slide motion from the upper chest to the abdominal area ten times.

The shanzhong (膻中, CV-17) cavity is commonly used to treat asthma, cough, bronchitis, chest pain and distention, dyspnea, lung abscess, pulmonary tuberculosis (TB), hematemesis, hemoptysis, insufficient lactation, breast abscess or mastitis, hypochondriac pain, facial pallor, palpitations, weak vocal cords, hiccups, esophageal constriction or dryness, anemia, and cardiac pain.

The jiuwei (鳩尾, CV-15) cavity is often used to treat pericarditis, chest pain, palpitations, asthma, lassitude, mental exhaustion, vomiting, acidity, hiccups, spasms of the diaphragm, gastralgia, cough, throat numbness and pain, migraine, pain of the abdominal skin (excess type), itching of the abdominal skin (deficiency type), hysteria, mania, and fear.

3. Sides of the Chest (胸側部)

After you finish the massage of the central chest area, focus on the side of your chest.

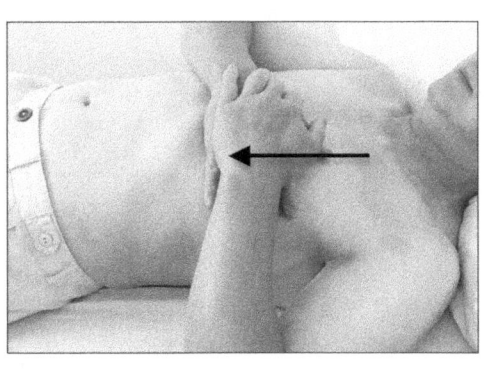

First use your two palms to push downward from the upper left chest to the waist area ten times.

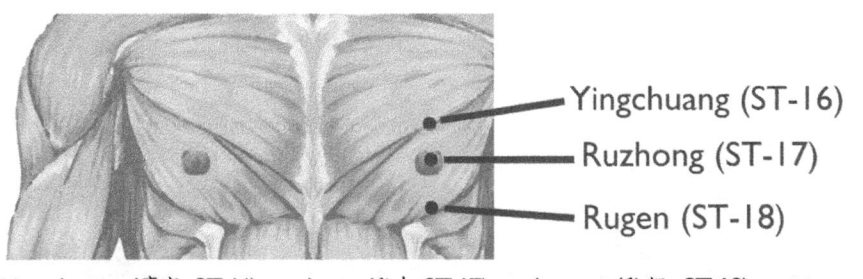

Yingchuang (膺窗, ST-16)
Ruzhong (乳中, ST-17)
Rugen (乳根, ST-18)

Yingchuang (膺窗, ST-16), ruzhong (乳中, ST-17), and rugen (乳根, ST-18) cavities.

Next use your index, middle, and ring fingers to press and vibrate the yingchuang (膺窗, ST-16), ruzhong (乳中, ST-17), and rugen (乳根, ST-18) cavities for ten seconds. Rest for a few seconds, and repeat the pressing vibration.

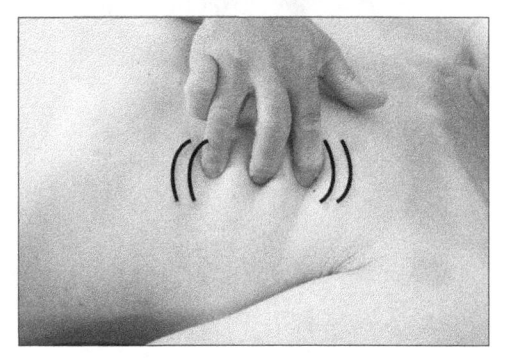

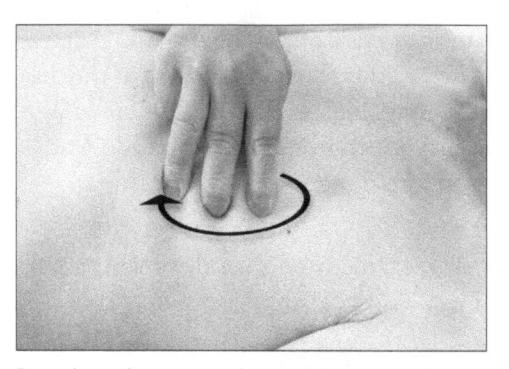

Rest for a few seconds, and then use the same fingers to rub the cavities in a circular motion for ten seconds. Rest for a few seconds, and repeat the circular rubbing massage for another ten seconds.

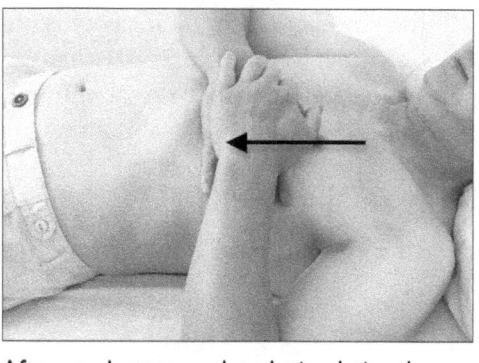

After you have completed stimulating these three cavities, repeat the pushing downward process ten times.

Finally, switch the entire massage procedure to your right chest area.

These three cavities—yingchuang (膺窗, ST-16), ruzhong (乳中, ST-17), and rugen (乳根, ST-18)—always work together in Chinese medicine and qigong massage. They can be used to alleviate chest fullness and pain, cough, bronchitis, asthma, insufficient lactation, mastitis, breast lumps, and prolonged menstruation.

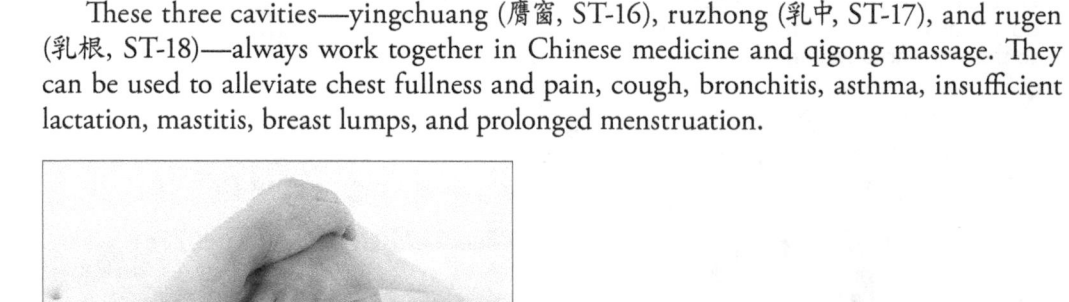

Finally, use the fingers of your right hand to push from the center to the left side of your chest, following the ribs ten times. Rest for a few seconds and repeat. Then use the fingers of the left hand to repeat the same pushing action to your right rib cage area.

4. Stomach and Abdominal Areas (胃部、小腹)

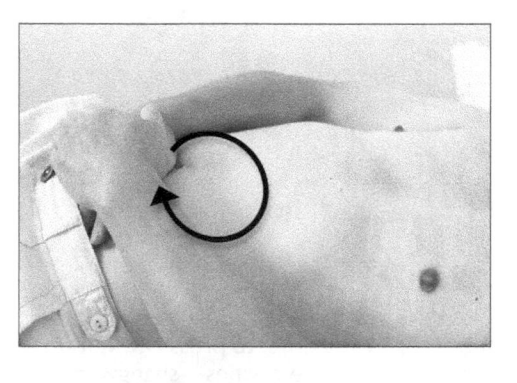

Overlap your palms, and gently circle the entire abdominal area ten times, following the direction of the bowel system. That means you will be circling in a clockwise direction.

It is important to follow the bowel system. If you reverse the direction, it is not releasing but nourishing. Circling in the reverse direction may cause constipation.

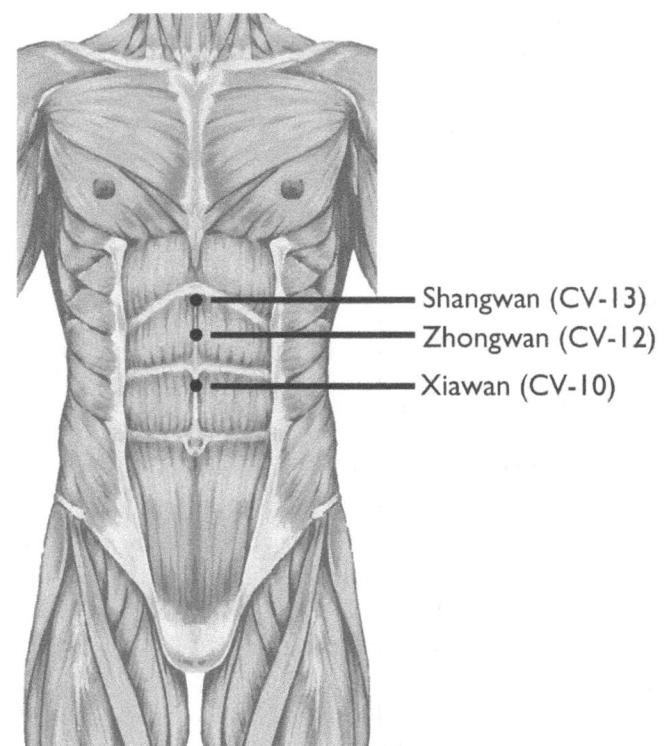

Shangwan (CV-13)
Zhongwan (CV-12)
Xiawan (CV-10)

Shangwan (上脘, CV-13), zhongwan (中脘, CV-12), and xiawan (下脘, CV-10) cavities.

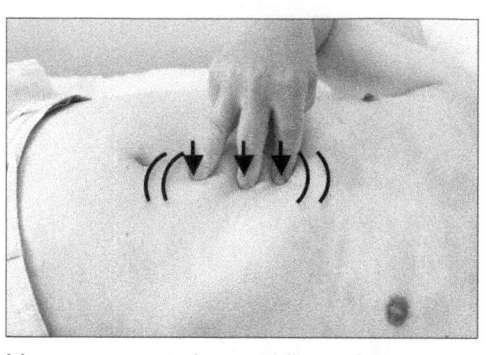

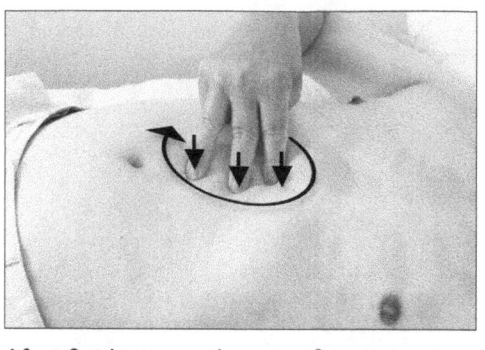

Next use your index, middle, and ring fingers, one at a time, to press and vibrate the following three cavities—shangwan (上脘, CV-13), zhongwan (中脘, CV-12), and xiawan (下脘, CV-10)—from the top cavity to the bottom. Rest for a few seconds, and repeat from the top cavity to the bottom.

After finishing, use the same fingers, one at a time, to rub each cavity in a circular motion in the direction of the bowel system. Rub the top one for ten seconds, and then move to the next cavity. After finishing all three, go back to the top one, and repeat the same circular rubbing process one more time.

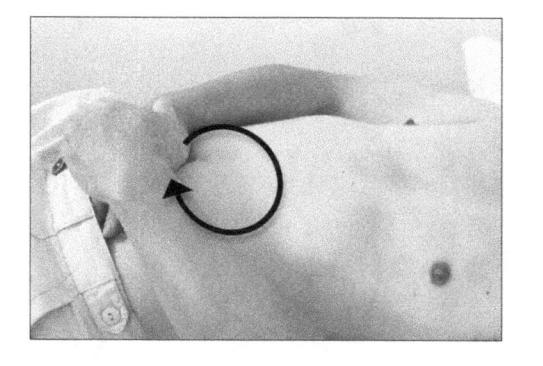

Finally, use both palms again to circle the entire abdominal area ten times, following the bowel system.

The treatments for these three cavities are very similar because they are related to one another and are all in the conception vessel, down the centerline of the front of the torso.

Specifically, the shangwan (上脘, CV-13) cavity is used to treat abdominal pain and distention, ulcers, morning sickness, stomach and epigastric pain, jaundice, hiccups, vomiting, cough with excessive sputum, excessive salivation, diarrhea, anorexia, bronchitis, seizures, insanity, palpitations, anxiety, and chest pain.

The zhongwan (中脘, CV-12) cavity can relieve abdominal pain and distention, all gastric diseases, nausea and vomiting, diarrhea, constipation, borborygmus, intestinal abscess, jaundice, dysentery, diabetes, childhood nutritional impairment, anorexia, ulcers, epigastric pain and distention, morning sickness, acid regurgitations, hiccups, gastroptosis or other organ prolapse, dizziness or vertigo, sinusitis, restless fetus, pulmonary TB, headache, hypertension, madness, Wei syndrome, emaciation, and weak limbs.

The xiawan (下脘, CV-10) cavity can be used to treat gastritis, duodenal ulcer, dysentery, abdominal pain, abdominal masses, borborygmus, diarrhea, anorexia, vomiting, and hematuria.

5. Groin Area (下陰部)

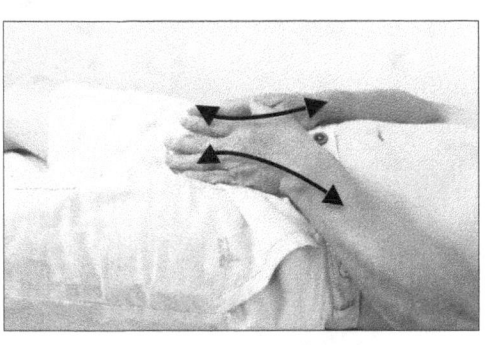

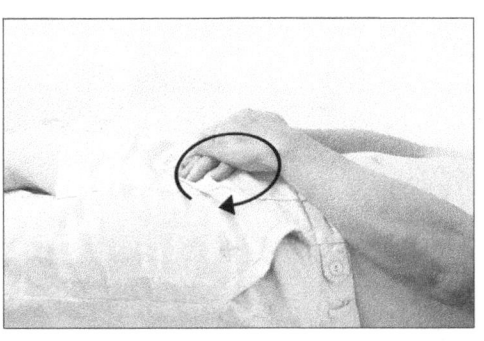

Use the edge of both hands, the pinky side, to rub and gently push the area between your abdomen and inner hip joint areas. Rub these areas for thirty seconds.

Next overlap your palms, and rub in a circular motion the area above the groin. Rub in one direction for thirty seconds, and then change direction for another thirty seconds.

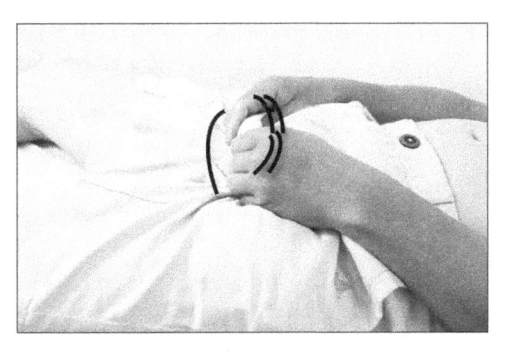

Next, for males, use both hands to gently massage the testicles for one minute. For females, use the base section of your thumbs to press, and rub the area above the ovaries. Rub in one direction for thirty seconds, and then change to the other direction for thirty seconds.

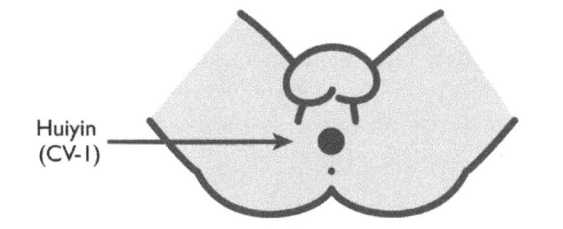

Huiyin (會陰, CV-1) cavity.

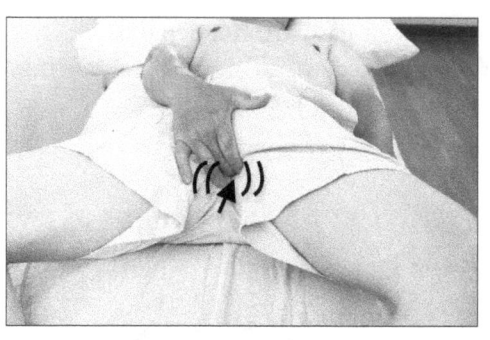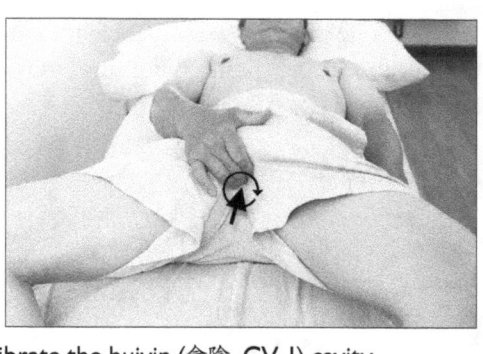

Finally, use your middle finger to gently press and vibrate the huiyin (會陰, CV-1) cavity (perineum) for thirty seconds, and then follow with circular rubbing motion for another thirty seconds.

The huiyin (會陰, CV-1) is known to treat all diseases of the perineal area, uterovaginal or rectal prolapse, genital or perineal swelling and pain, pruritus vulva, vaginitis, cold scrotum, itching, irregular menstruation, dysmenorrhea, amenorrhea, impotence, spermatorrhea, hemorrhoids, prostatitis, dysuria, urinary retention, night perspiration, hysteria, insanity, melancholia, coma, and also for reviving consciousness such as for drowning victims.

III. Lower Back and Hips (背腰、臀部) (彎膝)

There are two positions used to massage the lower back and hips. One is facing upward, and the other is facing sideways. Each position has its advantages and disadvantages. Therefore, you may choose either position. Naturally, if you have time, you may use both positions one after the other.

The advantages of the facing-upward position are as follows:

- The torso is more relaxed. In this case, you can reach a deeper level of relaxation.
- You can easily use your body's weight to generate massage pressure either for vibration or circular rubbing.

The disadvantage of the facing-upward position is as follows:

- You will not be able to use two common techniques used for stimulation—that is, hitting and slapping.

The advantage of the facing-sideways position is as follows:

- You can use two common techniques for stimulation—that is, hitting and slapping the cavity.

The disadvantages of the facing-sideways position are as follows:

- You can become tired more easily because you have to use your arms and hands to generate pressure. Naturally, this will make your body tenser as well.
- The torso is tenser in the sideways position than when facing upward, especially the lower back.

Facing Upward

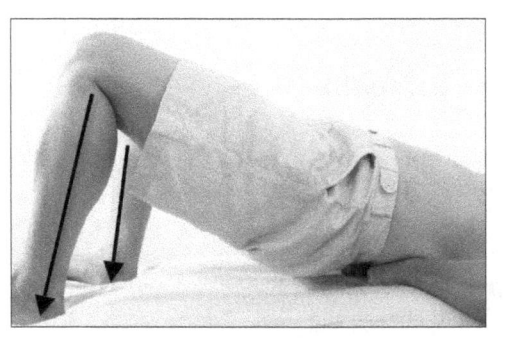

Lie facing upward with your knees bent. Use your legs to adjust how much pressure you would like to apply to the area or cavity.

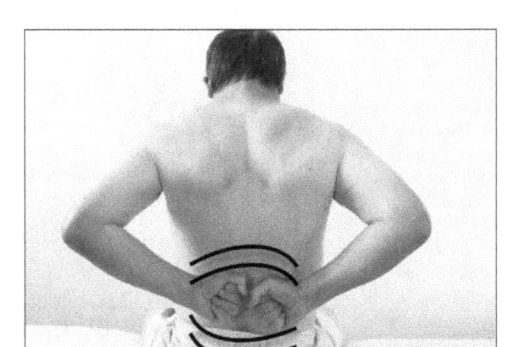

To stimulate the cavity, you may use the base knuckle of your index finger or the base knuckles of all your fingers.

The stimulation can be generated by pressing with vibration or by circular rubbing motions. As mentioned before, pressing with vibration can penetrate deeper, while circular rubbing motions can bring the stagnant qi to the surface and spread it.

There are ten cavities that are important for stimulation. You should follow the order from the top to the bottom so the qi can be led downward, especially if you have a history of lower back tension or pain.

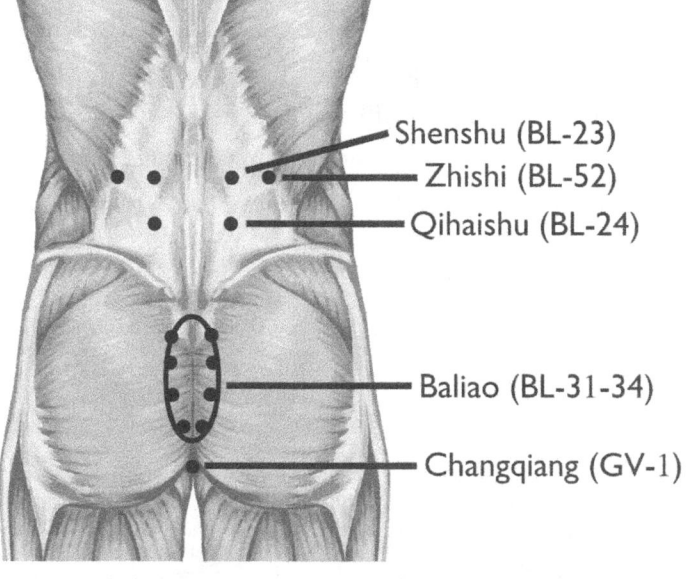

Shenshu (腎俞, BL-23), qihaishu (氣海俞, BL-24), zhishi (志室, BL-52), baliao (八髎, BL-31-34) (仙骨), and changqiang (長強, GV-1) (尾閭) cavities.

1. Shenshu (腎俞, BL-23)

The shenshu cavity is used to treat kidney, bladder, and urinary diseases; sexual problems; impotence; spermatorrhea; leukorrhea; irregular menstruation; infertility; premenstrual syndrome; amenorrhea; dysmenorrhea; genital pain; nephritis; cystitis; ascites; edema; kidney stones; lower back pain and muscular strain; knee pain; anemia; alopecia (hair loss); weakness and lassitude; asthma; diarrhea; indigestion; deafness; tinnitus; blurred vision; optic nerve atrophy; forgetfulness; anxiety and palpitations; and fear.

2. Qihaishu (氣海俞, BL-24)

This cavity can be used to treat lower back pain and stiffness, knee pain, hemorrhage, irregular menstruation, uterine bleeding, and weak or painful lower extremity.

3. Zhishi (志室, BL-52)

This cavity is commonly used for all genitourinary diseases, dysuria, spermatorrhea, urethral pain, painful urinary dysfunction, infertility, impotence, prostatitis, nephritis, anemia, edema, nocturnal emission, cystitis, incontinence, lower back pain, hypochondriac pain, nausea, vomiting, swelling of the genitalia, fear, poor memory, anxiety, poor concentration, and renal colic.

4. Baliao (八髎, BL-31-34) (仙骨)

There are eight cavities on the sacrum, four on each side. These cavities are used to treat urogenital diseases, dysuria, retention of urine, irregular menstruation, leukorrhea, dysmenorrhea, ovarian cyst or inflammation, spermatorrhea, orchitis, eczema of the perineum, peritonitis, diarrhea, constipation, lower back pain, stiffness and sciatica, foot numbness, anal fissure, uterovaginal prolapse, and bleeding hemorrhoids.

5. Changqiang (長強, GV-1) (尾閭)

This cavity is also called the tailbone. It can be used to treat hemorrhoids, painful and bloody hemorrhoids, rectal prolapse, ulcerative colitis, diarrhea, constipation, anal fissure, fecal incontinence, anal pain, itchiness and numbness, sacral pain and stiffness, scrotal eczema, spermatorrhea due to fright, pruritus vulvae, extreme nervousness, seizures, convulsions, depression, fatigue and lassitude, stiffness of the spine, heaviness of the head, and shaking of the head.

Massaging the following two cavities serve the purpose of opening up the connection junctions between the lower back and the legs. Furthermore, by stimulating these two cavities, you will be able to lead the stagnant qi in the lower back downward.

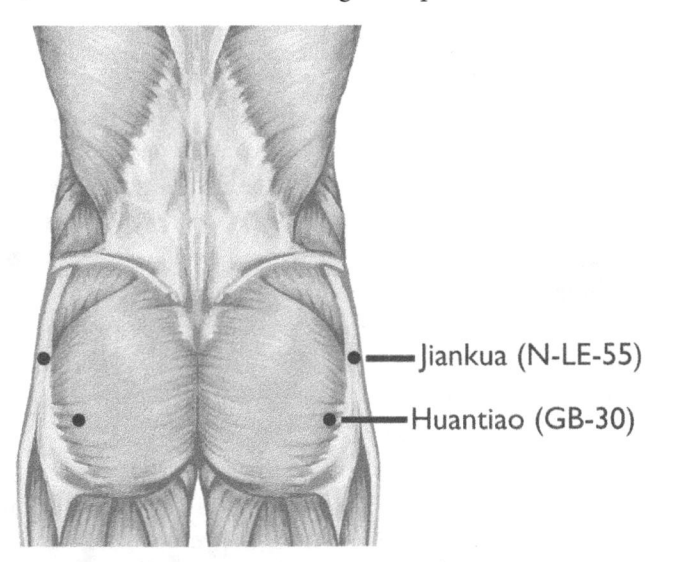

Huantiao (環跳, GB-30) and jiankua (健胯, N-LE-55) cavities.

6. Huantiao (環跳, GB-30)

This cavity can be used to treat hip joint inflammation, sprain and pain, sciatica, thigh muscular spasm, lower abdominal and lower back pain, leg paralysis, leg qi disorder, hemiplegia, urticaria, neurasthenia, and edema.

7. Jiankua (健胯, N-LE-55)

The last cavity you should stimulate on the torso is the jiankua (健胯, N-LE-55). This cavity is known for treating hemiplegia, paraplegia, hip pain, and thigh pain.

Facing Sideways

There are a couple of options for you to continue:

1. You may continue to the limbs.
2. You may want to add additional slapping and hitting massage on the same cavities listed above.
3. You may want to skip the facing-upward massage. Instead, go straight to the facing-sideways massage.

In the facing-sideways massage, simply follow the same stimulating procedures as above, except with additional slapping and hitting stimulation. Finish one side first, and then change to the other side.

IV. Limbs (四肢)

Before we continue on to limbs massage, you should know a few things. The external side of the limbs is considered yang while the inner side is considered yin. Yang's energy is manifested energy, and thus you may apply more power in the massage on the external side. The inner side of the limbs is considered yin and is more sensitive. Thus, the power you use for massage on the inner side must be gentler and softer.

When you massage beginning from the torso and then following the limbs outward, it is considered releasing the energy (洩, xie). If you reverse the direction, beginning from the limbs and massaging inward toward the torso, it is considered a nourishing process (補, bu). If you are not sick, it is usually better to release the energy and keep the energy moving instead of applying the nourishing technique, which slows down the releasing process.

The structure of the arms and legs are somewhat similar. This means that the cavities located on the arms often correspond to the cavities on the legs. If you are able to stimulate the corresponding cavities on the arms and legs at the same time, you will feel that the stimulation and circulation of the energy will be more balanced. In addition, if you are able to massage the arms and legs at the same time, you can also save half the time.

There are three cavities on the limbs that are considered the most important cavities for health and longevity: hegu (合谷, LI-4), zusanli (足三里, ST-36), and sanyinjiao (三陰交, SP-6). From the experience of many Chinese doctors and qigong practitioners, it has been verified that massaging these three cavities often maintains the body's qi circulation to a very healthy state.

In Chinese medical society, it is said that there are four major cavities for treating diseases: zusanli (足三里, ST-36), weizhong (委中, BL-40), lieque (列缺, LU-7), and hegu (合谷, LI-4). These four cavities and their usage in treatment are often remembered by a poem that is commonly known to all Chinese medical doctors: "For stomach and abdomen problems, be aware of zusanli. For waist and back problems, seek weizhong cavity. If there is problem on the head, then lieque must be located. When the face and mouth have problems, use hegu to solve the problem."[1]

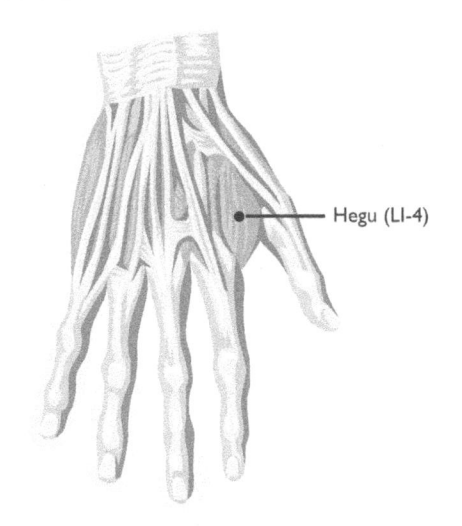

Hegu (合谷, LI-4) cavity.

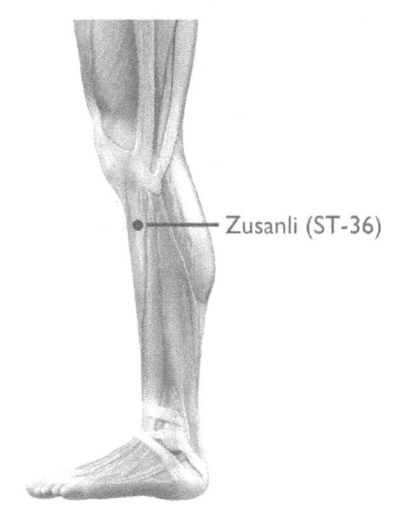

Zusanli (足三里, ST-36) cavity.

1. "肚腹三里留，腰背委中求，頭項尋列缺，面口合谷收。"

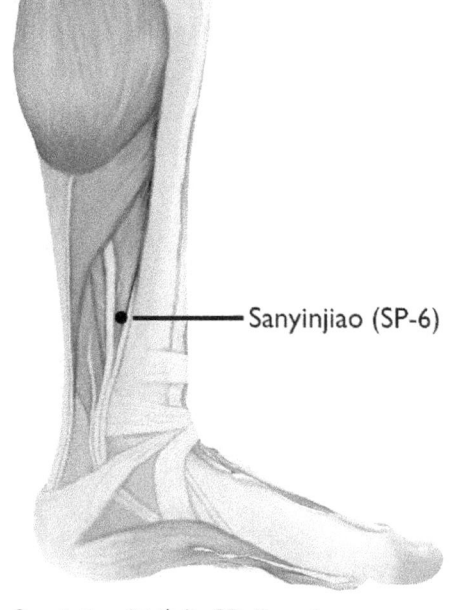

Sanyinjiao (三陰交, SP-6) cavity.

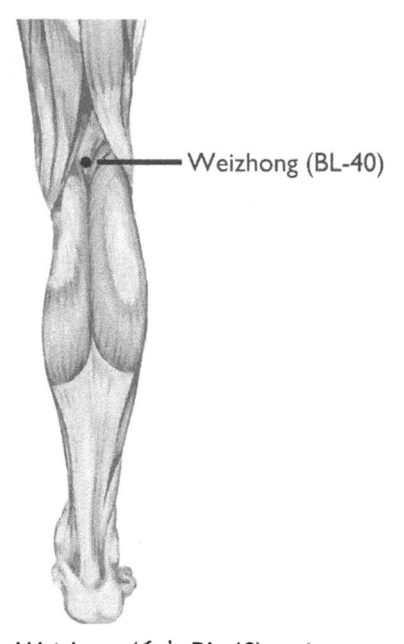

Weizhong (委中, BL-40) cavity.

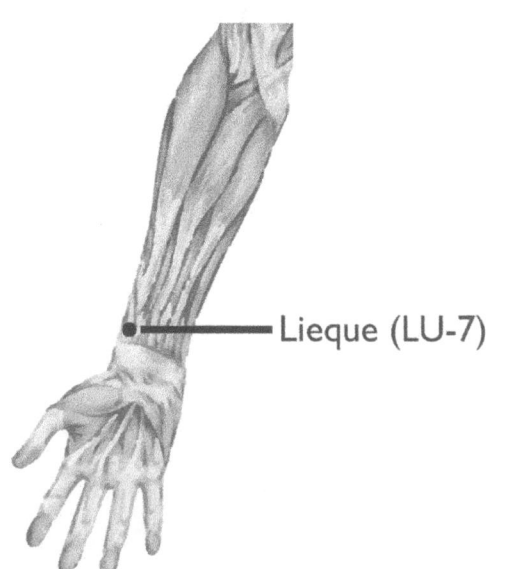

Lieque (列缺, LU-7) cavity.

External Limbs (Yang Side)

The following massages use corresponding cavities of the arms and legs.

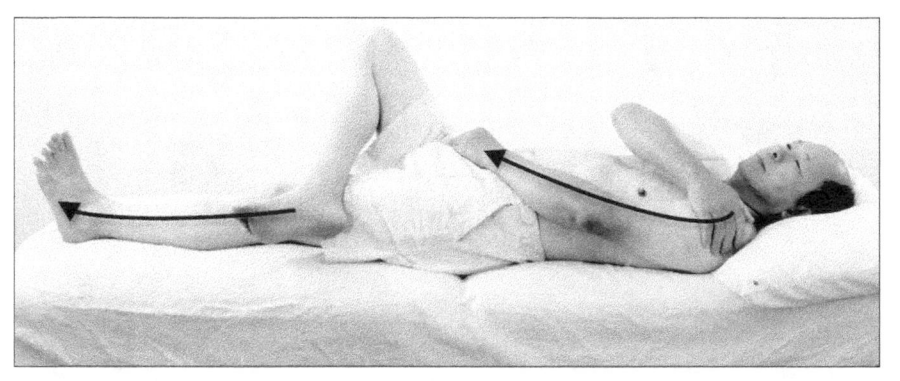

Use your right hand to push downward from the external side of the left upper arm to the left hand. Simultaneously, use the external side of your right ankle to push downward from the external side of your left thigh to the left foot. Repeat ten times.

The power applied should not cause too much pain. A comfortable stimulating pain is the right feeling. If the pain is too significant, you may cause the leg to be too tense and the qi circulation more stagnant. After you complete ten times of pushing, next stimulate these cavities in the following order.

1. Binao (臂臑, **LI-14**) ←→ **Fengshi** (風市, **GB-31**)

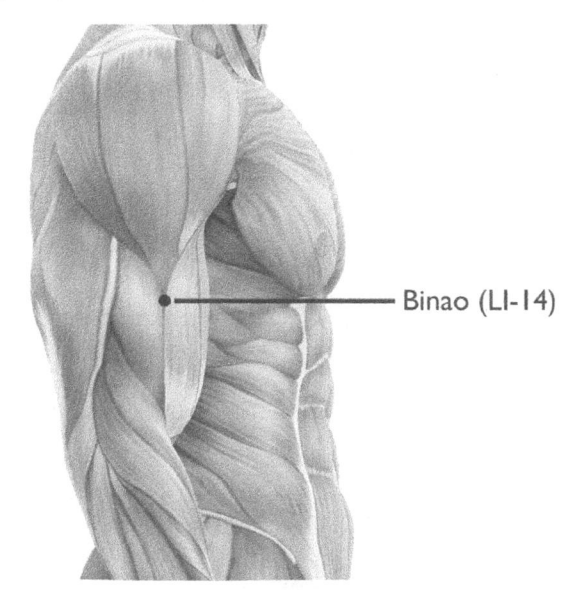

Binao (LI-14)

Binao (臂臑, LI-14) cavity.

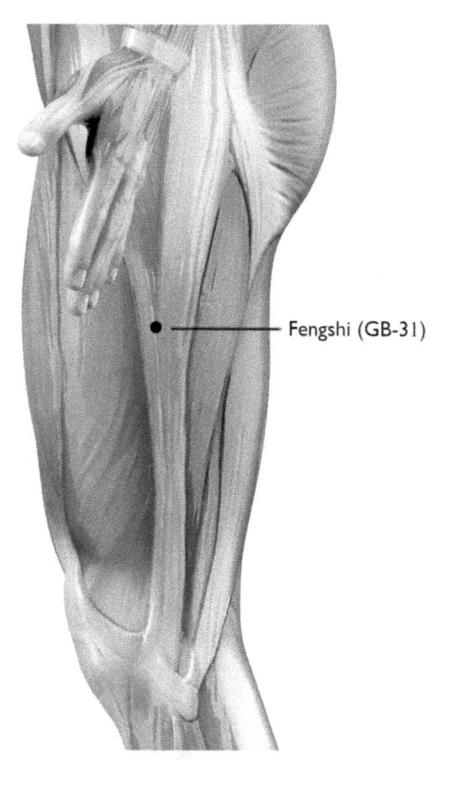

Fengshi (風市, GB-31) cavity.

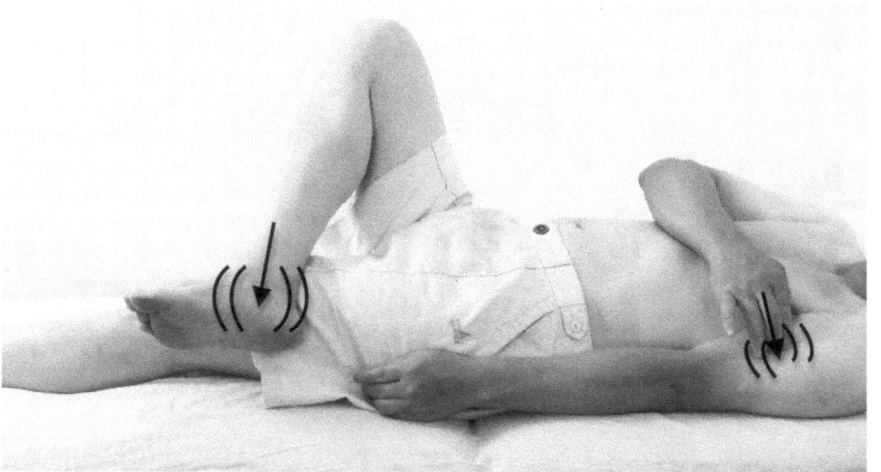

Use your index and middle fingers to press and vibrate the binao (臂臑, LI-14) cavity for ten seconds. While doing so, use your heel to press and vibrate the fengshi (風市, GB-31) cavity for ten seconds. Rest for a few seconds, and then stimulate them again for another ten seconds. Again, rest for a few seconds, and repeat.

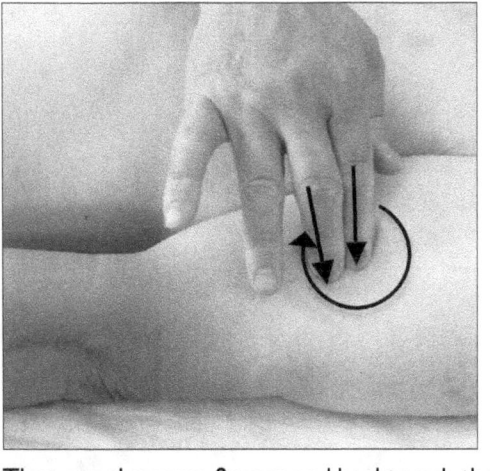
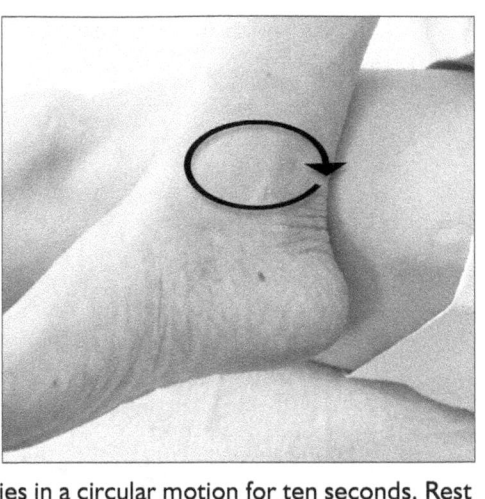

Then use the same fingers and heel to rub the cavities in a circular motion for ten seconds. Rest for a few seconds, and repeat.

The binao (臂臑, LI-14) cavity can be used to treat pain in the shoulder and arm, paralysis of the arm, stiffness of the neck and nape, eye diseases, conjunctivitis, myopia, goiter, and scrofula.

The fengshi (風市, GB-31) cavity is commonly used to treat thigh and knee weakness, leg qi disorder, lower back pain and sciatica, unilateral itching of the whole body, urticaria, herpes zoster, hemiplegia, red and swollen eyes, and pruritus.

2. Quchi (曲池, LI-11) ←→ Xuehai (血海, SP-10)

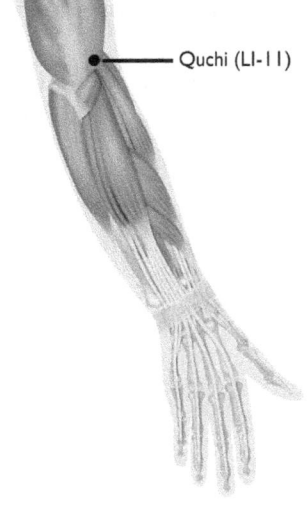
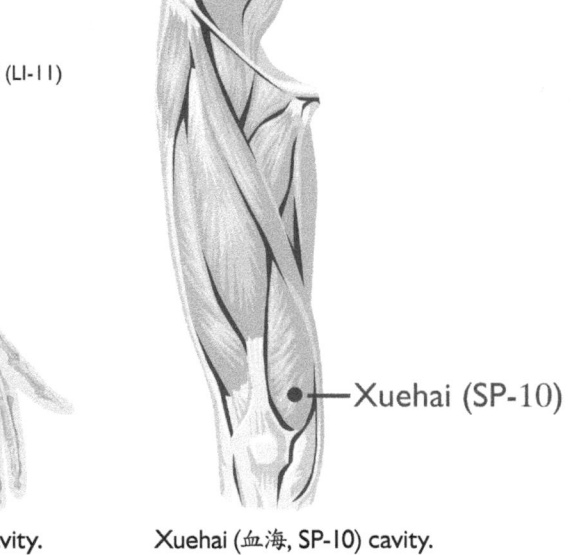

Quchi (曲池, LI-11) cavity.   Xuehai (血海, SP-10) cavity.

Next repeat the same stimulating process for the quchi (曲池, LI-11) and xuehai (血海, SP-10) cavities.

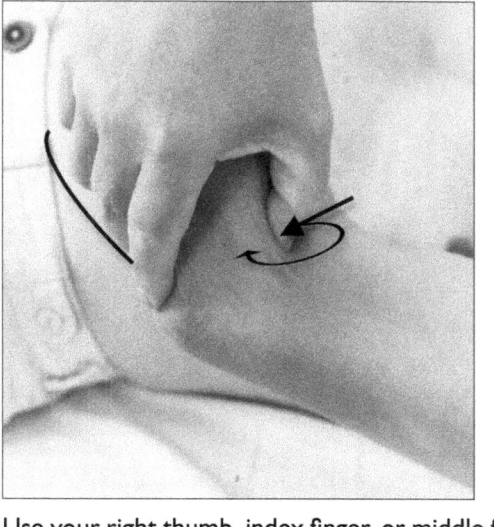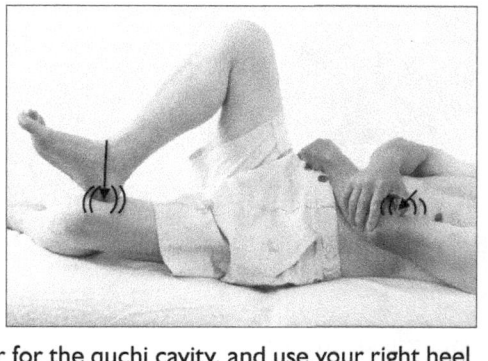

Use your right thumb, index finger, or middle finger for the quchi cavity, and use your right heel to stimulate the xuehai cavity with press vibration and circular rubbing.

The quchi (曲池, LI-11) cavity is commonly used to treat all febrile diseases, fever, sore throat, malaria, hemiplegia, pain and motor impairment of the shoulder, arm and elbow pain, swelling and pain of the knee, headache, dizziness, redness, swelling and pain of the eye, blurred vision, toothache, irregular menstruation, painful urine, common cold, convulsions, hypertension, rubella, eczema, urticaria, erysipelas, abdominal pain, vomiting, diarrhea, constipation, abdominal pain, bronchitis, chest pain, goiter, depressive psychosis and madness, and scrofula.

The xuehai (血海, SP-10) cavity can be used to treat excessive menstrual bleeding, all blood disorders, all skin diseases due to heat or heat toxin in the blood, blood in the urine, restless fetus, vaginal pruritus, herpes zoster, anemia, eczema, boils and carbuncles, orchitis, and allergies.

3. Shousanli (手三里, LI-10) ←→ Zusanli (足三里, ST-36), Yanglingquan (陽陵泉, GB-34)

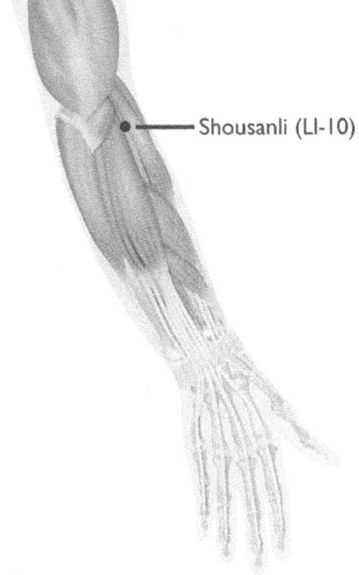

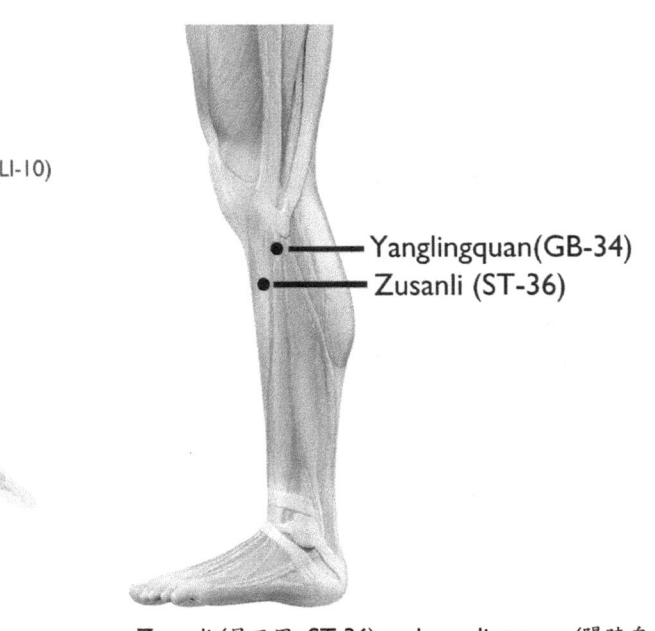

Shousanli (手三里, LI-10) cavity.

Zusanli (足三里, ST-36) and yanglingquan (陽陵泉, GB-34) cavities.

Next massage the shousanli (手三里, LI-10) cavity on the arm and the corresponding two cavities on the legs—zusanli (足三里, ST-36) and yanglingquan (陽陵泉, GB-34)—which are located near each other.

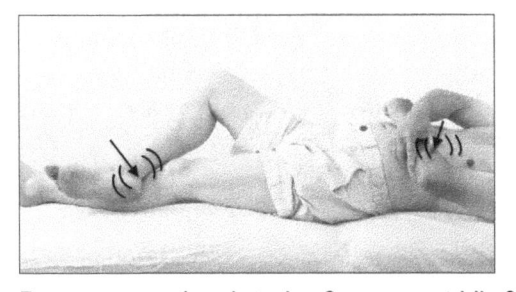

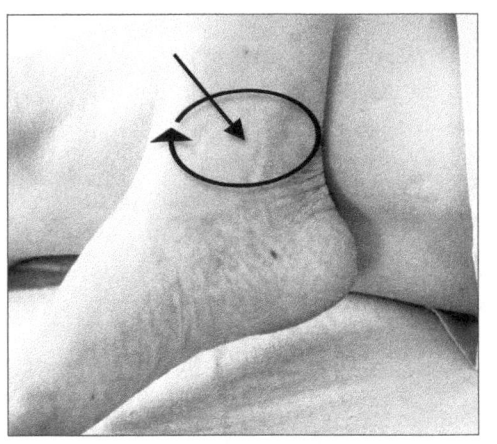

First use your thumb, index finger, or middle finger to press and vibrate the shousanli cavity while using the external anklebone (lateral malleolus) to press and vibrate the zusanli cavity for ten seconds. Rest for a few seconds, and repeat.

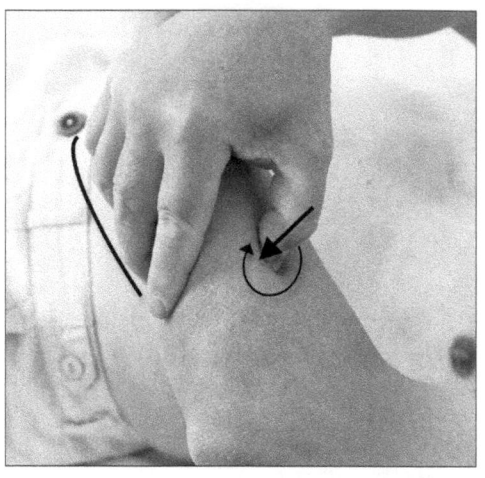

Next stimulate these two cavities by rubbing in a circular motion for ten seconds. Rest for a few seconds, and repeat.

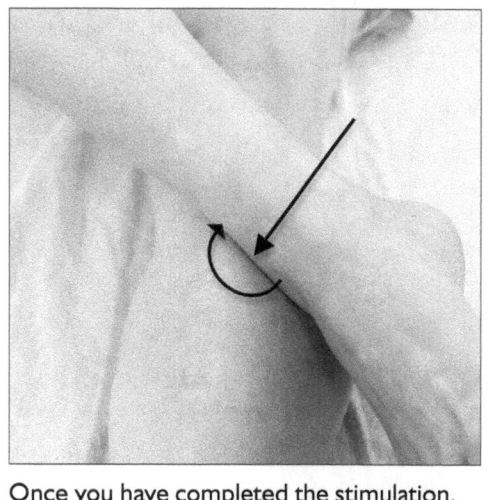

Once you have completed the stimulation, repeat the same process except changing the cavity you stimulate from zusanli to yanglingquan.

It is known that the shousanli (手三里, LI-10) cavity can be used to treat facial paralysis, arm paralysis, cramps and edema, shoulder pain, hemiplegia, abdominal distention, diarrhea, vomiting, goiter, breast abscess, swelling of submandibular region, and arm pain.

The zusanli (足三里, ST-36) cavity is a well-known and popularly used cavity both in acupuncture and qigong. It is recognized as one of the three major cavities that can be used for health and longevity. The zusanli cavity can be used for treating stomach and spleen diseases, anorexia, intestinal abscess, bloody dysentery, abdominal masses, digestive ulcers, colitis, appendicitis, enteritis, pancreatitis, nausea, diarrhea, constipation, insomnia, general weakness, asthma, nephritis, restless fetus, skin diseases, urticaria, eczema, breast abscess, allergies, anemia, dizziness, vertigo, headache, sinusitis, tinnitus, hypertension, hemiplegia, insufficient lactation, and eye diseases.

The yanglingquan (陽陵泉, GB-34) cavity can be used to treat biliary diseases; jaundice; cholecystitis; hepatitis; hypochondria; intercostal, axillary, and shoulder pain and distention; biliary colic; liver cirrhosis; bitter taste in the mouth; swelling of the mouth, tongue, face, and head; erysipelas of the lower body; headache; hypertension; hyperacidity; leg qi imbalance; constipation; weak extremities; spasms; sciatica; hip and knee pain and inflammation; fright; insanity; and madness.

4. Yangchi (陽池, TB-4) ←→ Jiexi (解谿, ST-41)

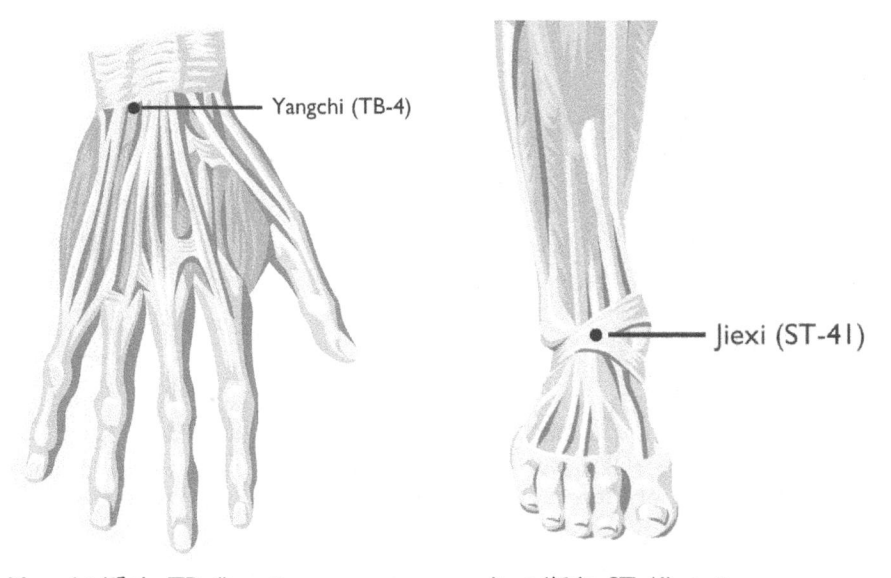

Yangchi (陽池, TB-4) cavity.

Jiexi (解谿, ST-41) cavity.

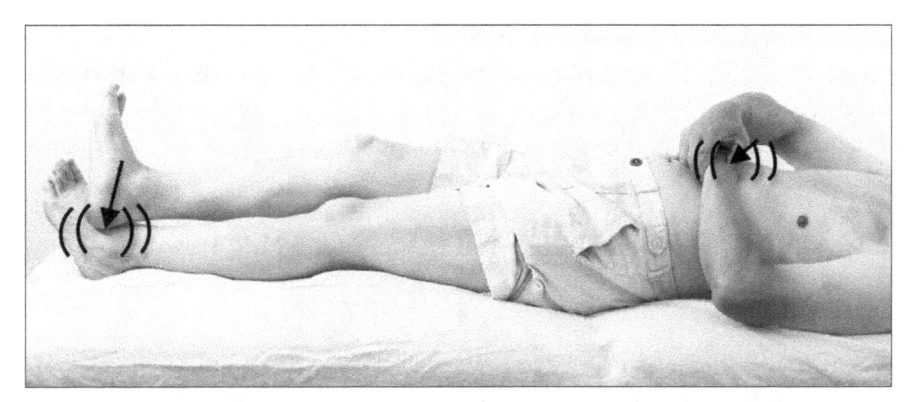

Next use your right thumb to press and vibrate the yangchi (陽池, TB-4) cavity on the left wrist joint while using your right heel to press and vibrate the jiexi (解谿, ST-41) cavity on the left ankle joint for ten seconds. Rest for a few seconds, and repeat for another ten seconds.

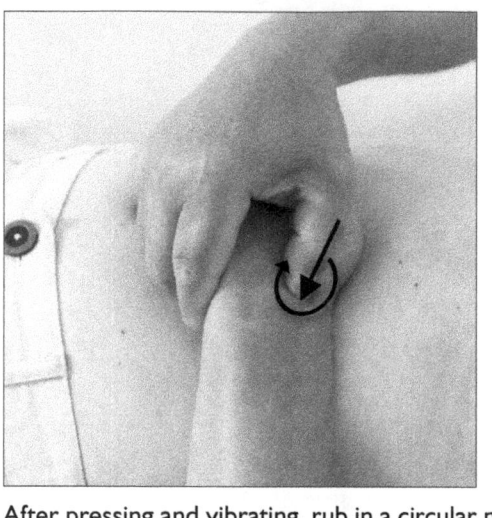
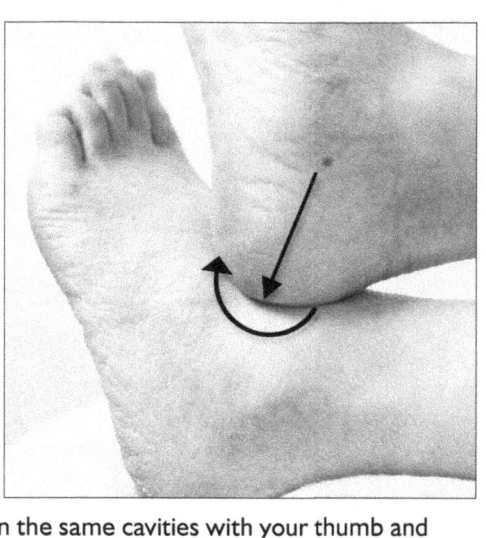

After pressing and vibrating, rub in a circular motion the same cavities with your thumb and heel for ten seconds. Rest for a few seconds, and repeat the same stimulating process for another ten seconds.

The yangchi (陽池, TB-4) cavity can be used to treat problems such as wrist pain and weakness, malaria, tidal fever, tonsillitis, conjunctivitis, fatigue, dry mouth and throat, diabetes, melancholy, and general weakness.

The jiexi (解谿, ST-41) cavity can be used to treat headache, dizziness, edema of the face, mouth pain, eye disease, abdominal distention, constipation, delirium, seizures, mania, incoherent speech, ankle pain and sprain, foot drop, red eyes with headache, fright, and toothache.

5. Hegu (合谷, LI-4) (虎口, Hukou) ←→ Taichong (太衝, LR-3)

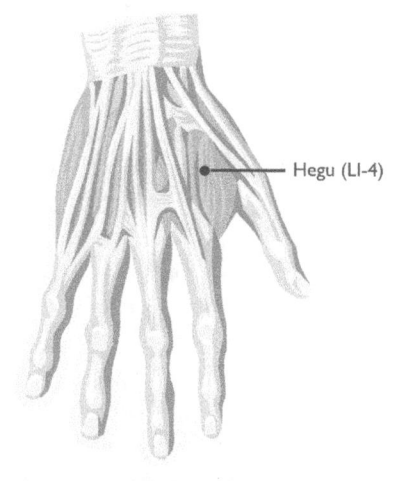
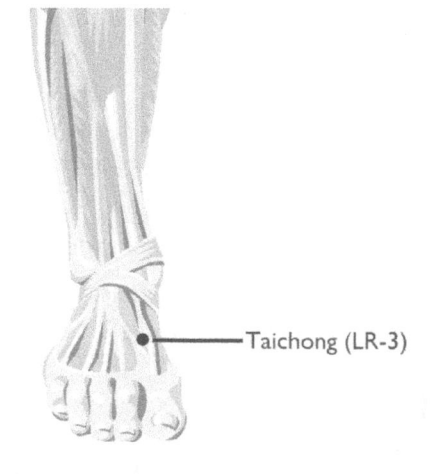

Hegu or hukou (合谷, LI-4) (虎口) cavity.

Taichong (太衝, LR-3) cavity.

Finally, stimulate the last two cavities of the external side of the limbs: hegu (合谷, LI-4) and taichong (太衝, LR-3). The hegu cavity is also called Tiger Mouth (虎口, kukou) by laypeople. As mentioned before, the hegu is one of the four major cavities commonly used in Chinese acupuncture.

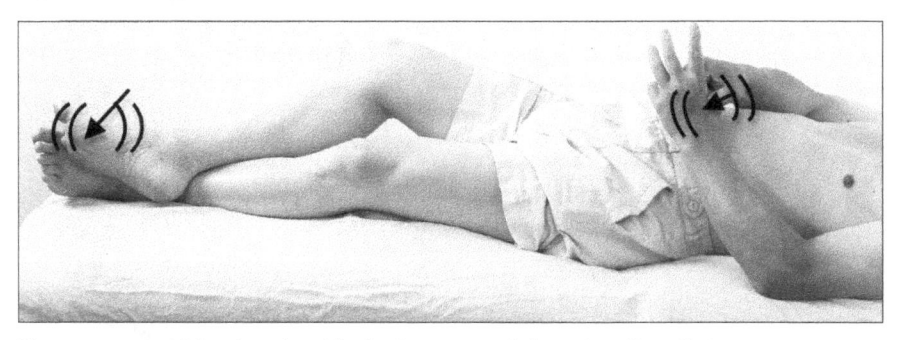

First use your right thumb with the leverage of the other four fingers to generate pressure on the hegu cavity on the left hand. Then vibrate it for ten seconds. While you are doing so, use the base of the little toe of the right foot to press and vibrate the taichong (太衝, LR-3) cavity on the left foot. Rest for a few seconds, and repeat.

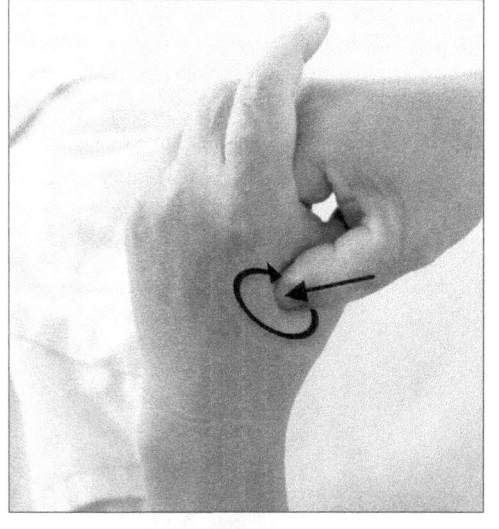 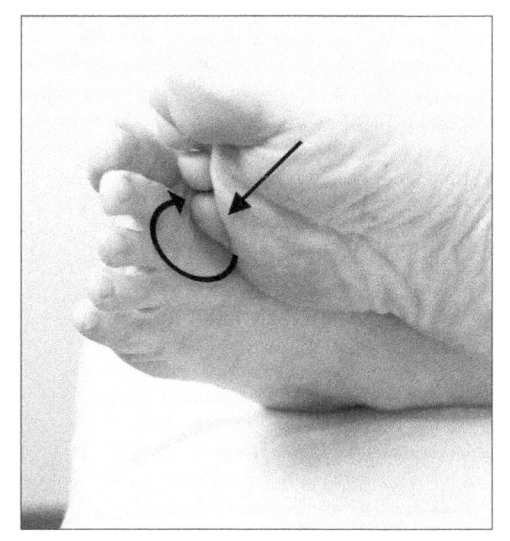

Then use your right thumb and the base of the little toe of the right foot to rub the cavities in a circular motion for ten seconds. Rest for a few seconds, and repeat the same process one more time.

The hegu (合谷, LI-4) (虎口, hukou) cavity can be used to treat eczema, erysipelas, trigeminal neuralgia, flu, common cold, mumps, amenorrhea, otitis media, urticaria, hemiplegia, chills, toothache, sneezing, headache, migraine, asthma, pruritis, bronchitis, diarrhea, appendicitis, constipation, abdominal pain, lymphangitis, furuncles, tetany, hysteria, tonsillitis, throat and tongue pain, voice loss, coma, fever, heatstroke, eye disorders, glaucoma, conjunctivitis, myopia, sudden blindness, difficult labor, and nasal disorders.

The taichong (太衝, LR-3) cavity treats all biliary diseases, hepatitis, jaundice (yang type), cholelithiasis, hyperthyroidism, hernia, menopausal and premenstrual syndrome (PMS), frigidity, dysuria, epigastric pain, constipation or diarrhea, hiccups, insomnia, nausea, vomiting, abdominal pain and distention, restless fetus, breast abscess, blood in the stool, glaucoma, red and painful eyes, trigeminal neuralgia, vertigo, temporal or vertical headache, temporomandibular joint pain, insufficient lactation, and mastitis.

After you have completed cavity stimulation of the entire left-side limbs, use your right hand and right ankle to push downward from the upper areas of the limbs to the hand and foot. In other words, repeat the same pushing process as described in the beginning of the limbs massage.

Naturally, after you have completed the massage for all your left external limbs, you should repeat the entire massage sequence for your right external limbs.

Inner Limbs (Yin Side)

Massage on the inner side of the limbs is very similar to massage of the external side of the limbs. The main difference is in the areas of the hand and leg used for massage. In addition, because the inner side of the limbs is more sensitive, the power used for massage is also different. It is important to remember that a comfortable level of pain is enjoyable and beneficial, while a significant level of pain will cause more tension and stagnation.

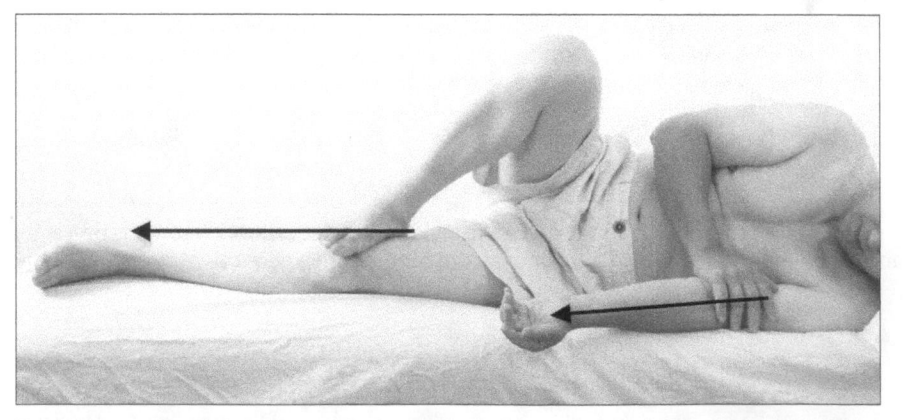

First use your right hand to push down from the inner side of the left upper arm toward the left hand and use the bottom of your right foot to push down from the inner side of the left thigh toward the left foot ten times.

After you complete ten repetitions of pushing, stimulate the next cavities in the following order.

1. Gongzhong (肱中, EX-UE-21) ←→ Jimen (箕門, SP-11)

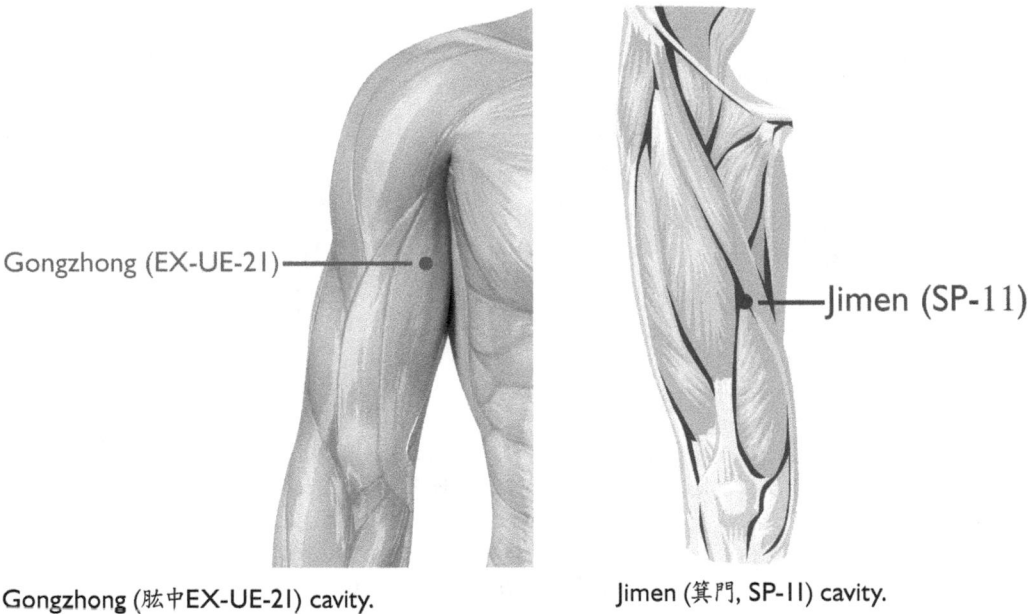

Gongzhong (肱中EX-UE-21) cavity.

Jimen (箕門, SP-11) cavity.

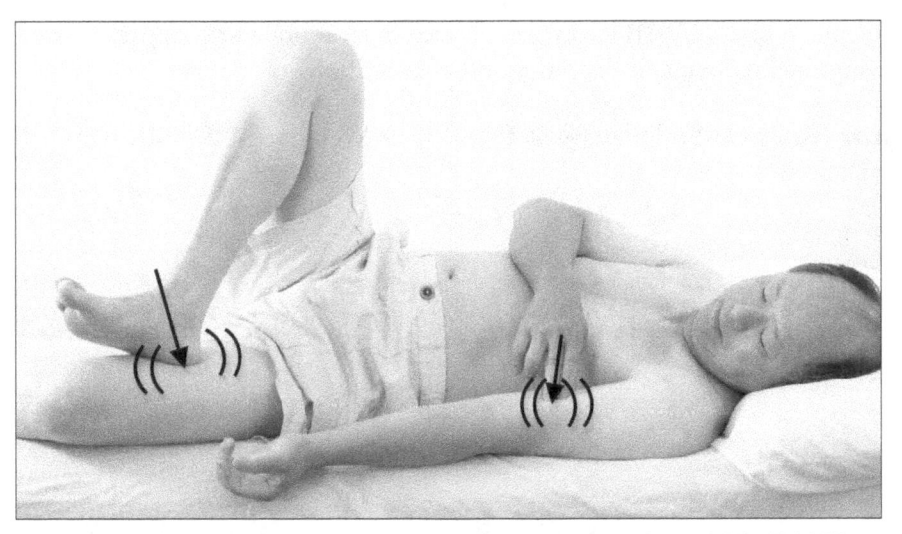

Use your right middle finger to press and vibrate the gongzhong (肱中, EX-UE-21) cavity on the left upper arm while using your right heel to press and vibrate the jimen (箕門, SP-11) cavity on the left thigh for ten seconds.

The inner side of your thigh is one of few most sensitive places in your body. If you find using the heel to stimulate jimen is too painful, you may simply use the bottom of your foot. Rest for a few seconds, and repeat the pressing and vibrating stimulation for another ten seconds.

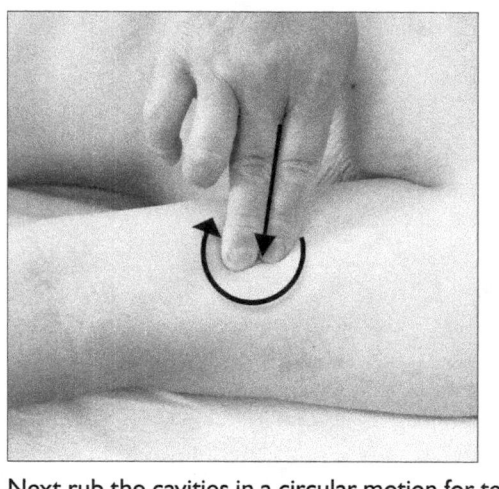 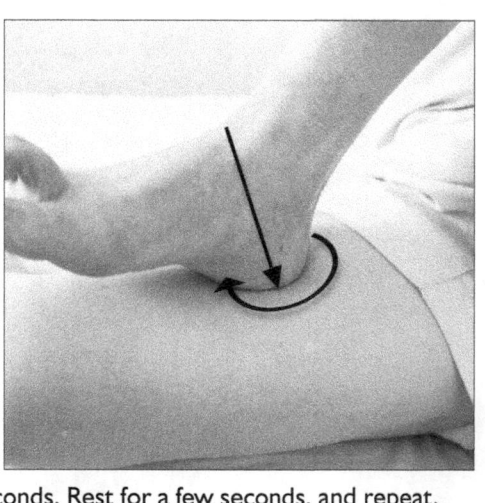

Next rub the cavities in a circular motion for ten seconds. Rest for a few seconds, and repeat.

The gongzhong (肱中, EX-UE-21) cavity is used to treat numbness of the upper limbs, difficulty in raising the arms, and weakness of the wrist. It is also recognized that massaging this cavity can help weight loss.

The jimen (箕門, SP-11) cavity can be used to treat bradyuria, enuresis, swelling pain in the inguinal region, and flaccidity of the lower limbs.

2. Chize (尺澤, LU-5), Quze (曲澤, PC-3) ←→ Weizhong (委中, BL-40)

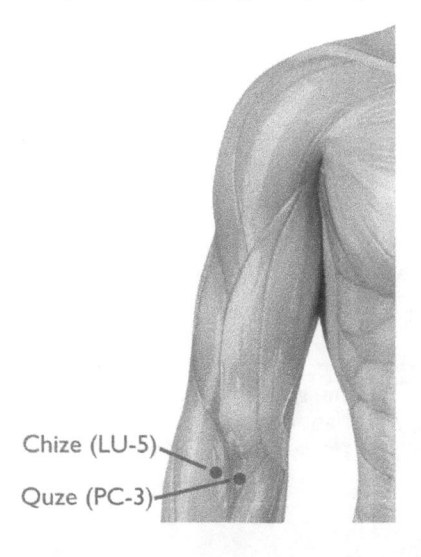

Chize (LU-5)
Quze (PC-3)

Chize (尺澤, LU-5) and quze (曲澤, PC-3) cavities.

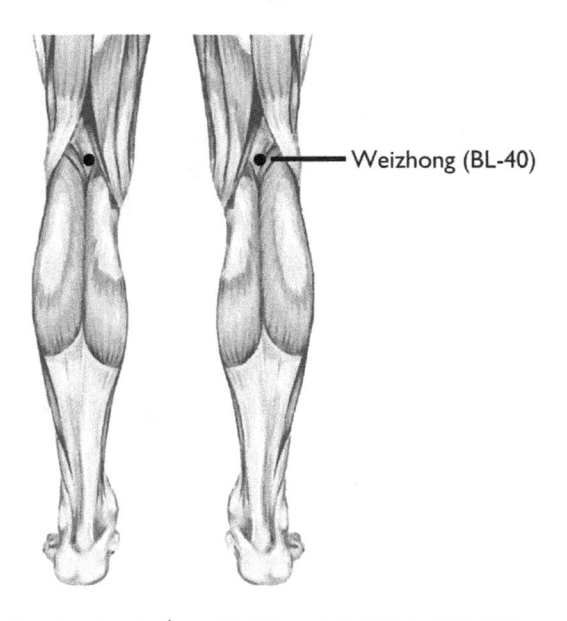

Weizhong (委中, BL-40) cavity.

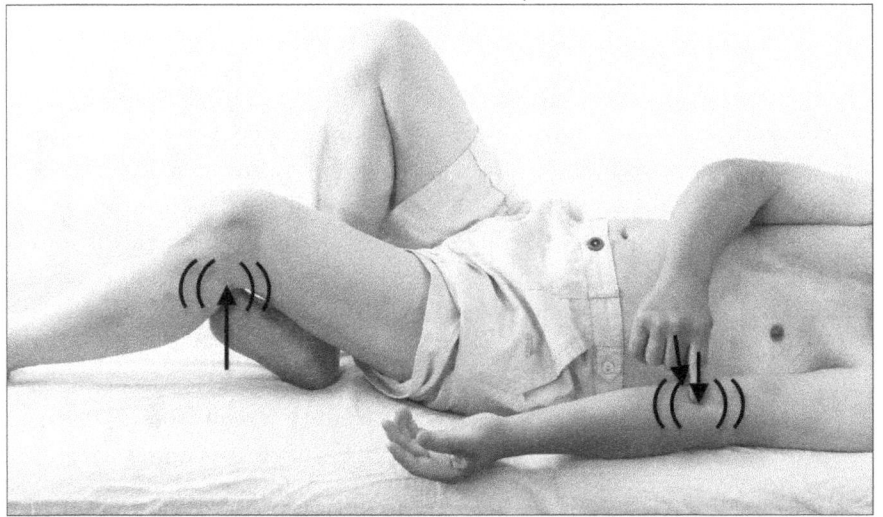

Next use your right index finger to press the chize (尺澤, LU-5) cavity and your right thumb on the quze (曲澤, PC-3) cavity on your left elbow joint and vibrate them for ten seconds. While doing so, position the tip of your right big toe on the weizhong (委中, BL-40) cavity in the center directly behind your left knee joint. The weight of the leg will provide the right pressure, and all you need to do is vibrate your left knee to stimulate this cavity. After ten seconds of pressing vibration, rest for a few seconds, and repeat the stimulation.

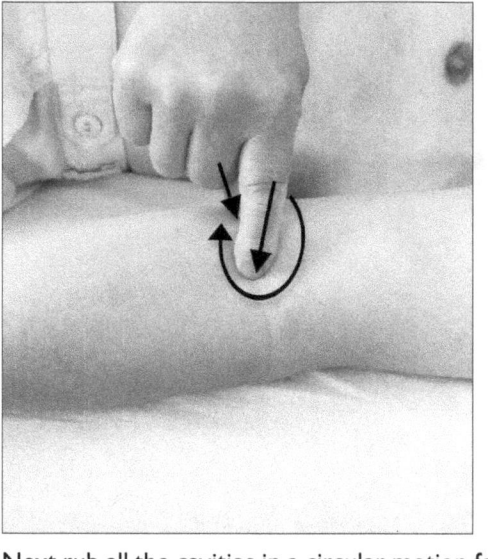
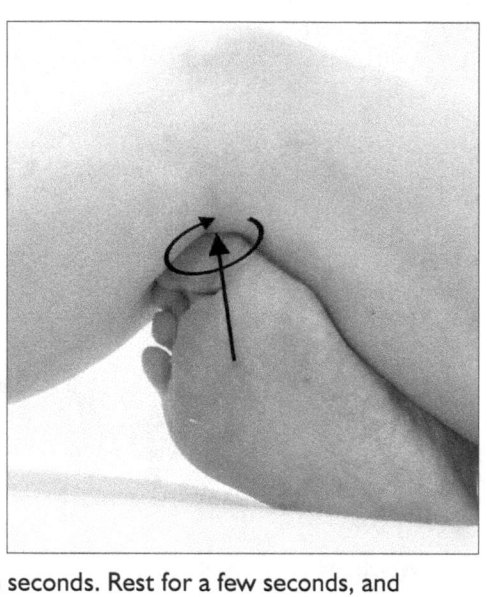

Next rub all the cavities in a circular motion for ten seconds. Rest for a few seconds, and repeat.

The chize (尺澤, LU-5) cavity is usually used to treat cough, asthma, bronchitis, chest fullness, hemoptysis, throat blockage, throat swelling, throat pain, dry mouth, thirst, fever, diabetes, Wei syndrome due to lung heat consumption, erysipelas, psoriasis, dry cough, renal pain, rigidity of the vertebral column, sneezing, and madness.

The quze (曲澤, PC-3) cavity can be used for treating stifling sensation in the chest, palpitations, irritability, myocarditis, cough, dyspnea, hand tremors, Parkinson's disease, perspiration of the head and neck, heatstroke, gastroenteritis, vomiting, stomachache, diarrhea with blood, erysipelas, urticaria, measles, sterility, and chorea.

It was mentioned earlier that the weizhong (委中, BL-40 [54]) cavity is one of the four major cavities that is commonly used for treating diseases. The weizhong cavity can be used for treating lower back pain, stiffness, and sciatica; lumbar sprain; herniated disc; heat- or sunstroke; skin diseases; eczema; psoriasis; furuncle; boils and carbuncles; herpes zoster; erysipelas; fever; spontaneous perspiration; acute abdominal pain; cystitis; dysuria; incontinence; diarrhea; convulsions; muscular spasm; knee pain and stiffness; epistaxis; bleeding hemorrhoids; alopecia; and loss of eyebrow hair.

3. Kongzui (孔最, LU-6) ←→ Yinlingquan (陰陵泉, SP-9)

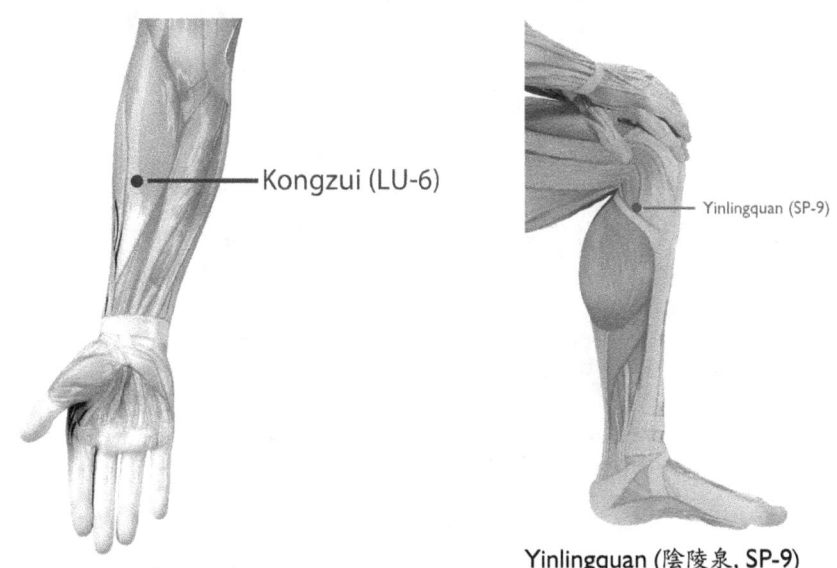

Kongzui (LU-6)

Yinlingquan (SP-9)

Kongzui (孔最, LU-6) cavity.

Yinlingquan (陰陵泉, SP-9) cavity.

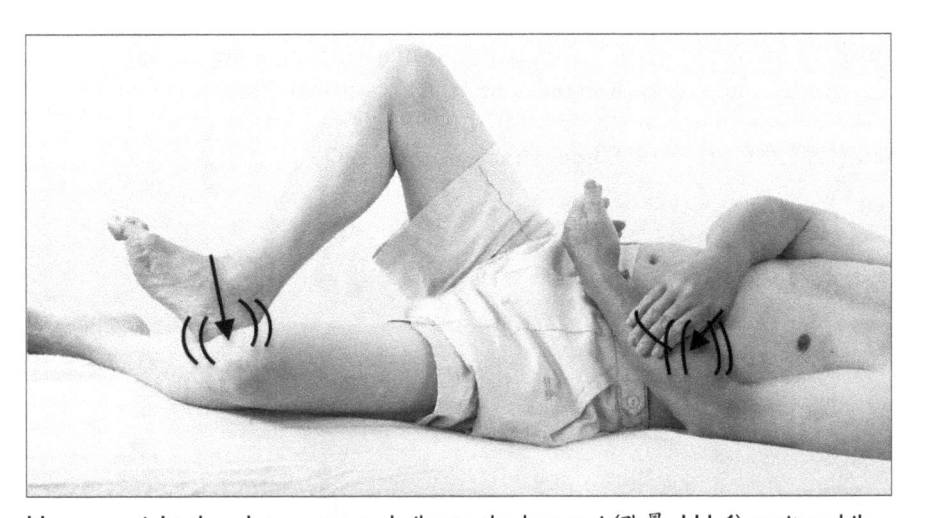

Use your right thumb to press and vibrate the kongzui (孔最, LU-6) cavity while using your right heel to press and vibrate the yinlingquan (陰陵泉, SP-9) cavity for ten seconds. Rest for a few seconds, and repeat the stimulation.

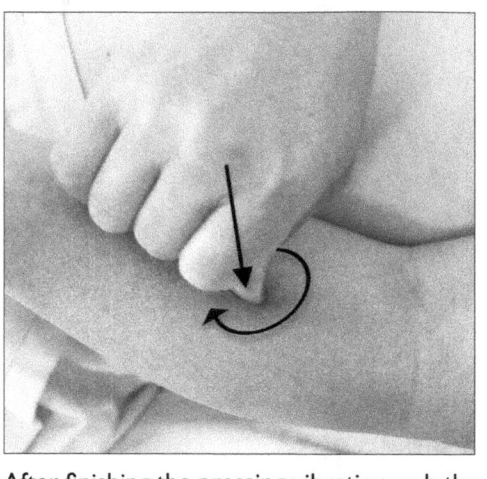 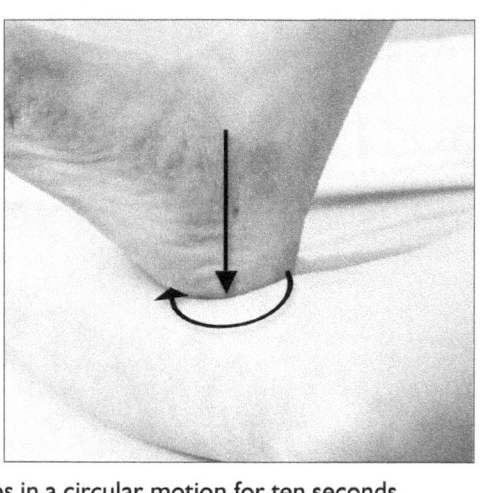

After finishing the pressing vibration, rub the cavities in a circular motion for ten seconds. Again, rest for a few seconds, and repeat the rubbing for ten seconds.

The kongzui (孔最, LU-6) cavity can be used to treat asthma, cough, bleeding, acute lung diseases, headaches, migraine, laryngitis, tonsillitis, skin diseases, hemoptysis, hemorrhoids, and pulmonary TB.

The yinlingquan (陰陵泉, SP-9) cavity is commonly used for treating edema, ascites, general urinary problems, cystitis, leukorrhea, urinary incontinence or retention, diarrhea, hepatitis, jaundice, nephritis, stomachache, and abdominal distention.

4. Ximen (郄門, PC-4) ←→ Chengshan (承山, BL-57)

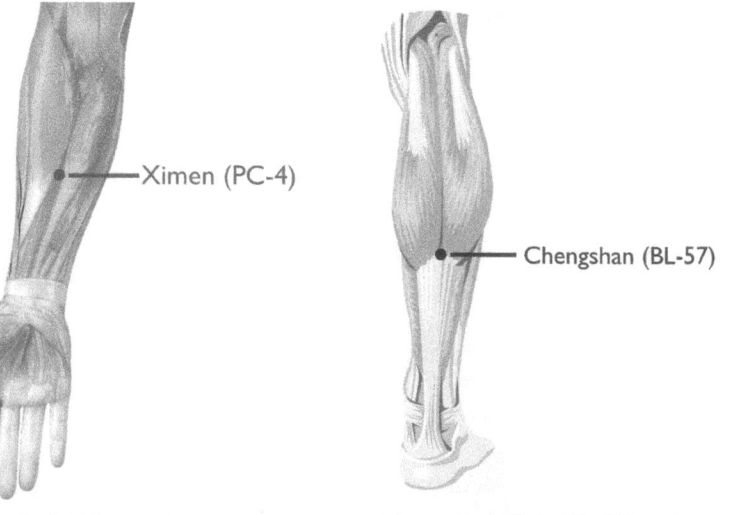

Ximen (郄門, PC-4) cavity.

Chengshan (承山, BL-57) cavity.

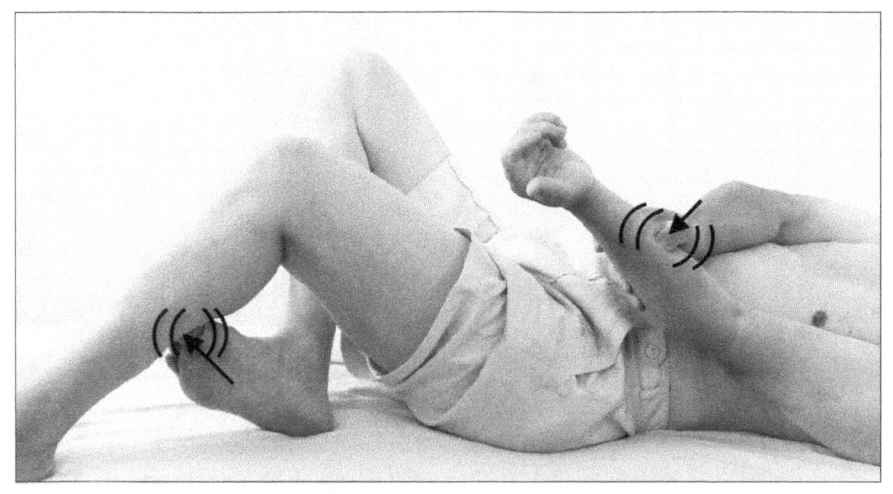

Use your right thumb to press and vibrate the ximen (郄門, PC-4) cavity on your left forearm while using the tip of your right big toe to press and vibrate the chengshan (承山, BL-57) cavity on your left leg for ten seconds. Rest for a few seconds, and repeat.

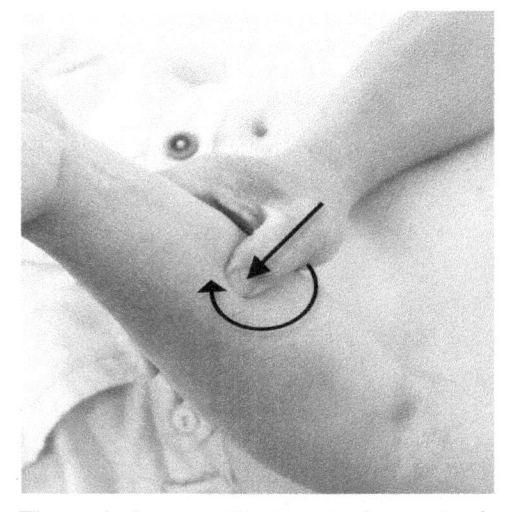 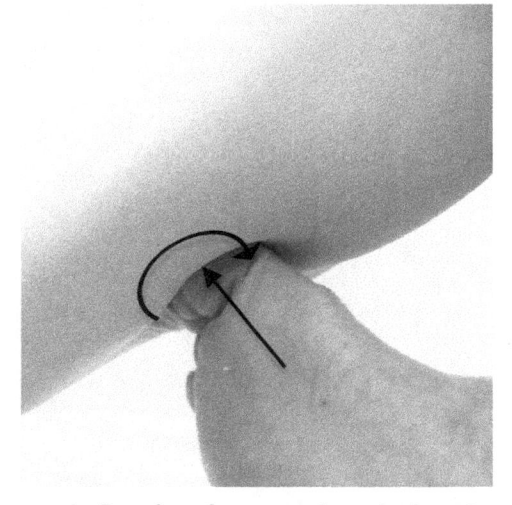

Then rub these cavities in a circular motion for ten seconds. Rest for a few seconds, and rub again.

The ximen (郄門, PC-4) cavity is known for treating rheumatic heart disease, angina pectoris, chest and heart pain, myocarditis, palpitations, tachycardia, diaphragmatic spasm, depression, fear of people, nervousness, forgetfulness, insomnia, melancholy, hemoptysis, epistaxis, nausea, and hemorrhoids.

The chengshan (承山, BL-57) cavity can be used to treat bleeding or painful hemorrhoids, anal prolapse, diarrhea, constipation, gastrocnemius muscle pain and spasm, sciatica, hernia, urethritis, abdominal pain, tremors, convulsions, and lockjaw.

5. Neiguan (內關, PC-6), Lieque (列缺, LU-7) ←→ Sanyinjiao (三陰交, SP-6)

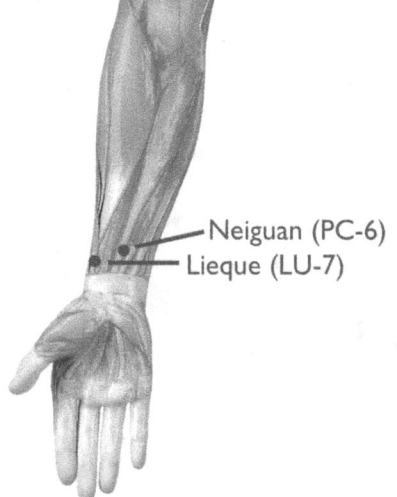

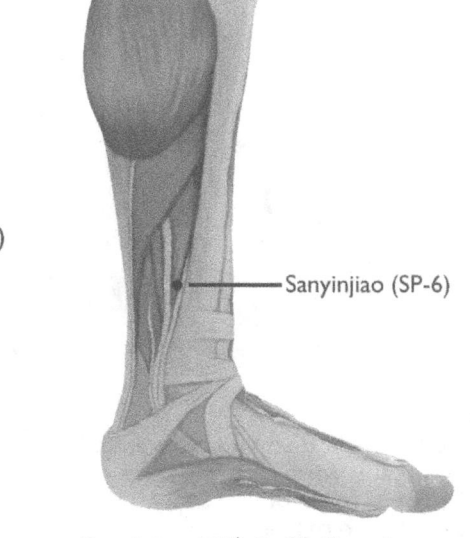

Neiguan (內關, PC-6) and lieque (列缺, LU-7) cavities.

Sanyinjiao (三陰交, SP-6) cavity.

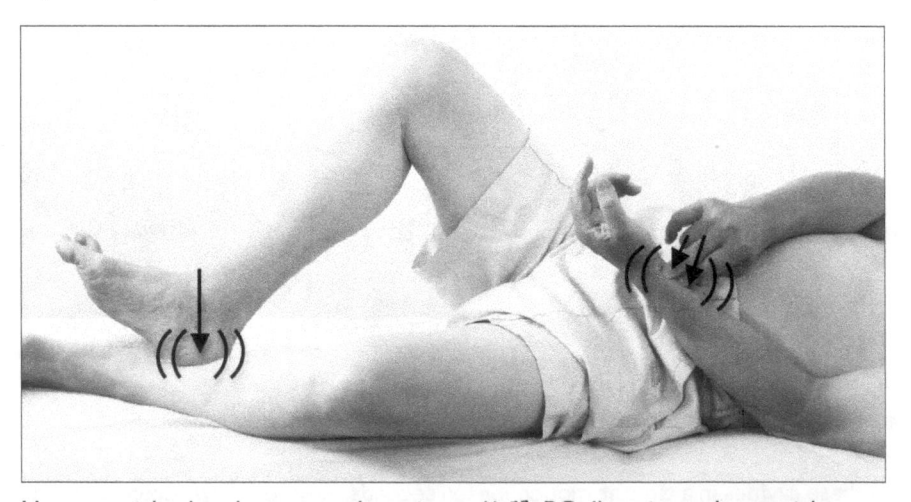

Use your right thumb to press the neiguan (內關, PC-6) cavity and your right index finger to press the lieque (列缺, LU-7) cavity on your left forearm, and vibrate them for ten seconds. While doing so, use your right heel to press and vibrate the sanyinjiao (三陰交, SP-6) cavity on your left leg. Rest for a few seconds, and repeat the stimulation for another ten seconds.

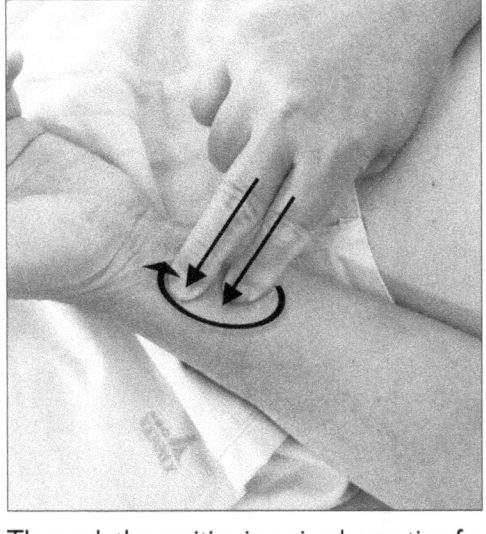
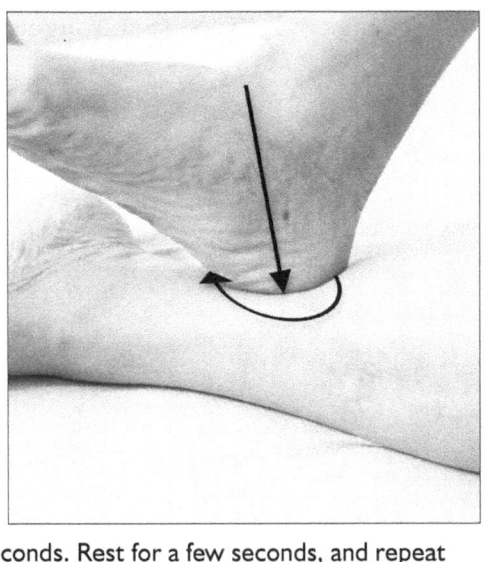

Then rub the cavities in a circular motion for ten seconds. Rest for a few seconds, and repeat for another ten seconds.

The neiguan (內關, PC-6) cavity can be used for treating cardiac and chest pain, rheumatic heart disease, hyperthyroidism, palpitations and anxiety, asthma, bronchitis, pertussis, dyspnea, nausea, morning sickness, vomiting, abdominal and gastric pain, hiccups, spasm of the diaphragm, malaria, dysentery, restless fetus, biliary diseases, jaundice, gallstones, pancreatitis, appendicitis, migraine, epigastric and hypochondriac pain and distention, irregular menstruation, fainting, coma and shock, seizures, hysteria, forgetfulness, and insomnia.

The lieque (列缺, LU-7) cavity is commonly used to treat wind-cold, stiff neck, facial paralysis, trigeminal neuralgia, urticaria, wind rash, hemorrhoids, dry and scaly skin, limbs edema, nasal problems, asthma, cough, sore throat, frontal and lateral headache, rhinitis, influenza, burning urination, hematuria, spermatorrhea, penile pain, pain and itching along the conception vessel (ren mai, 任脈), pain and inflammation of the umbilicus, semiparalysis of the face, toothache, weakness and pain in the wrist, hysterical laughter, yawning, loss of memory, and cold back and limbs.

As mentioned earlier, the sanyinjiao (三陰交, SP-6) cavity is one of the three most important cavities for health and longevity. This cavity is often used to treat all diseases of the lower abdomen, abdominal distention, diarrhea, leukorrhea, cloudy urination, eczema, urticaria, enuresis, dysuria, cystitis, urinary retention, weakness, dizziness, neurasthenia, insomnia, irregular menstruation, amenorrhea, dysmenorrhea, infertility, prolapse of uterus, difficult labor, leg qi imbalance, flatulence, hypertension, nephritis, prostatitis, impotence, organ prolapse, hernia, enlarged spleen, liver cirrhosis, and abdominal masses and tumors.

6. Laogong (勞宮, PC-8) ←→ Yongquan (湧泉, KI-1)

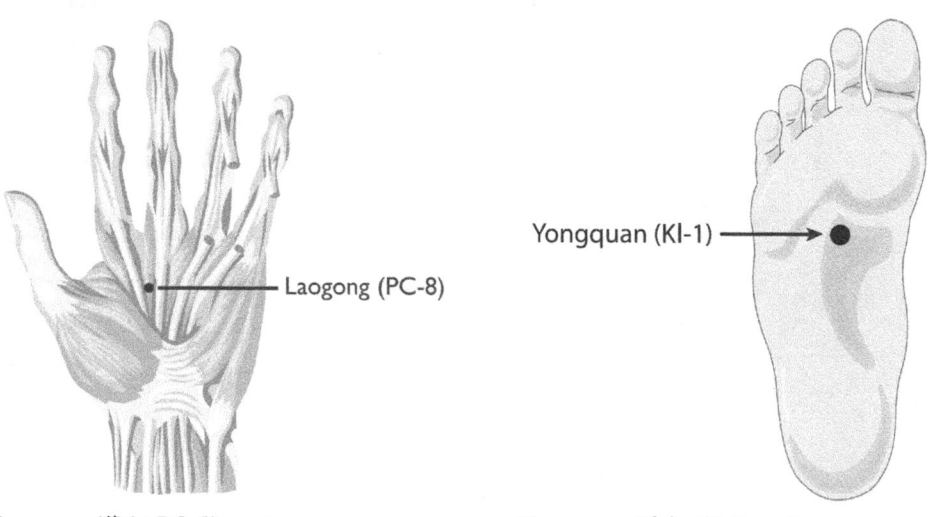

Laogong (PC-8)

Yongquan (KI-1)

Laogong (勞宮, PC-8) cavity.

Yongquan (湧泉, KI-1) cavity.

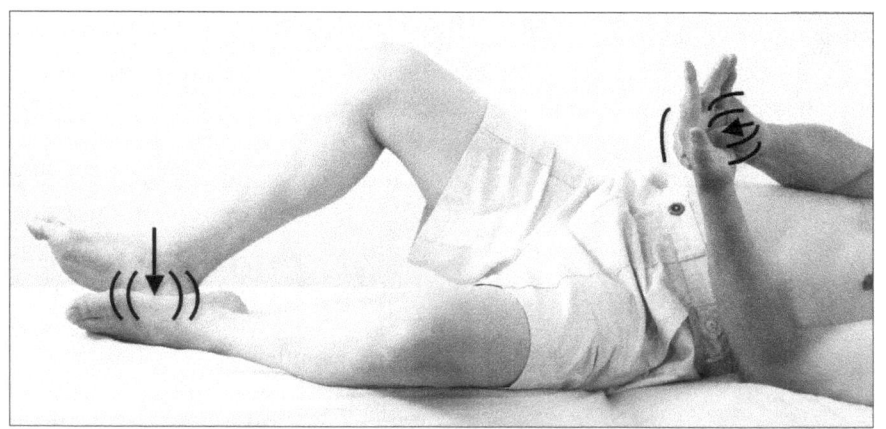

Use your right thumb to press and vibrate the laogong (勞宮, PC-8) cavity on your left palm while using your right heel to press and vibrate the yongquan (湧泉, KI-1) cavity on your left foot for ten seconds. When you use your thumb to press the laogong cavity, you may use the other four fingers as leverage to generate a good massage pressure. Rest for a few seconds, and repeat the pressing and vibration for another ten seconds.

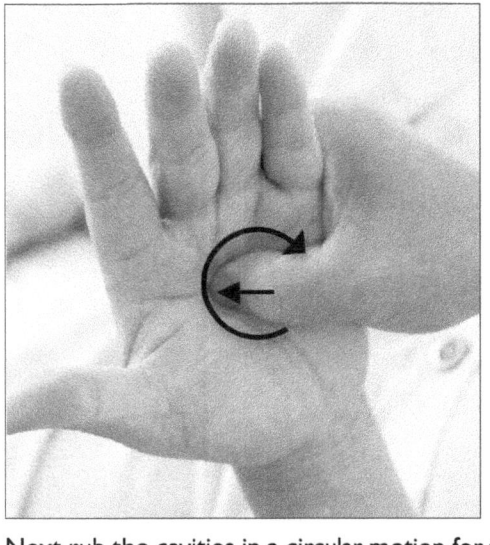 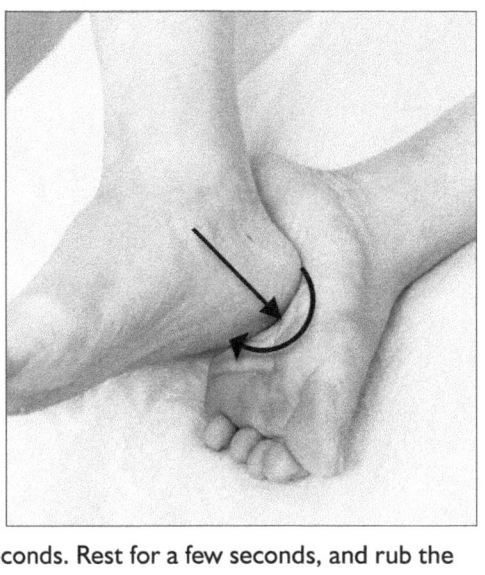

Next rub the cavities in a circular motion for ten seconds. Rest for a few seconds, and rub the cavities again.

After you finish all the cavity stimulations, push downward along the inner side of the limbs, from the upper arm toward the fingers, and from the upper thigh toward the toes, ten times. This completes the left-hand side of the limbs massage. Naturally, you should repeat the entire pushing and cavity-stimulation process on your right side.

The laogong (勞宮, PC-8) cavity is used to treat febrile diseases, epistaxis, gingivitis, halitosis, stomatitis, inability to swallow, chest and hypochondriac pain and fullness, excessive perspiration of the palms, fungal infections of the hands and feet, headache, thirst, blood in urine or stool, hemorrhoids, indigestion, wind stroke collapse, heatstroke, and incoherent speech.

The yongquan (湧泉, KI-1) cavity can be used for treating fainting, cerebrovascular accident, asphyxia (drowning), excessive sleepiness, dizziness, blurred vision, sore and swollen throat, dry mouth and tongue, aphonia, infertility, heat in the soles, edema, anorexia, borborygmus, kidney pain, scrotal inflammation, very red face, pain in the toes, and vertical headache.

After you have completed your massage of the entire body (except your upper back), lie down comfortably with a calm mind, keep your body as relaxed as possible, and breathe deeply and slowly for a few minutes. This will allow the qi to redistribute itself to a more balanced state. Then you can get up and resume your daily activities. If you massage right before you sleep, you may simply allow yourself to fall sleep.

Chapter 3: Qigong Theory Review

3-1. General Qigong Concepts

In this section, we will review the traditional concepts of qi and qigong. This can be helpful even if you have some qigong experience, and this is essential if you are a beginner. We will discuss the scope of qigong practice, the differences between external elixir (wai dan, 外丹) and internal elixir (nei dan, 內丹) qigong practice, and the differences between qigong schools in Chinese history. Then, in order to understand the practice concepts, the theories of yin-yang (陰陽) and kan-li (坎離) will be explained. Finally, we will summarize the relationship of qigong practice to health, longevity, and spiritual enlightenment.

1. Traditional Definition of Qi

In this subsection, we will first define the general concepts of qi, followed by the narrow concepts of qi. To understand the meaning of qigong practice, you must first have a clear idea of how qi is defined.

A General Definition of Qi 氣之廣義

Qi is the energy or natural force that fills the universe. The Chinese have traditionally believed that there are three major powers in the universe. These three powers (san cai, 三才) are heaven (tian, 天), earth (di, 地), and man (ren, 人). Heaven (the sky or universe) has heaven qi (tian qi, 天氣), the most important of the three, which is made up of the forces that the heavenly bodies exert on the earth, such as sunshine, moonlight, the moon's gravity, and the energy from the stars. In ancient times, the Chinese believed that heaven qi governed the weather, climate, and natural disasters. Chinese people still refer to the weather as heaven qi. Every energy field strives to stay in balance, so whenever heaven qi loses its balance, it tries to rebalance itself. Then the wind must blow, rain must fall, and even tornadoes or hurricanes become necessary in order for heaven qi to reach a new energy balance.

Under heaven qi is earth qi. It is influenced and controlled by heaven qi. For example, too much rain will force a river to flood or change its path. Without rain, plants will die. The Chinese believe that earth qi is made up of lines and patterns of energy as well as the earth's magnetic field and the heat concealed underground. These energies must also be in balance; otherwise, disasters such as earthquakes will occur. When the qi of the earth is balanced and harmonized, plants will grow, and animals will thrive.

Finally, within earth qi, each individual person, animal, and plant has its own qi field, which always seeks to be balanced. When any individual living thing loses its qi balance, it will sicken, die, and decompose. All natural things, including mankind and our human qi, grow within and are influenced by the natural cycles of heaven qi and earth qi. Throughout the history of qigong, people have been most interested in human qi and its relationship with heaven qi and earth qi.

In the Chinese tradition, qi can also be defined as any type of energy that is able to demonstrate power and strength. This energy can be electricity, magnetism, heat, or light. For example, electric power is called electric qi (dian qi, 電氣), and heat is called heat qi (re qi, 熱氣). When a person is alive, his body's energy is called human qi (ren qi, 人氣).

Qi is also commonly used to express the energy state of something, especially living things. As mentioned before, the weather is called heaven qi because it indicates the energy state of the heavens. When something is alive, it has vital qi (huo qi, 活氣); when it is dead, it has dead qi (si qi, 死氣) or ghost qi (gui qi, 鬼氣). When a person is righteous and has the spiritual strength to do good deeds, he is said to have normal qi or righteous qi (zheng qi, 正氣). The spiritual state or morale of an army is called energy state (qi shi, 氣勢).

You can see that the word *qi* has a wider and more general definition than most people think. It does not refer only to the energy circulating in the human body. Furthermore, the word *qi* can represent the energy itself, but it can also be used to express the manner or state of the energy. It is important to understand this when you practice qigong, so that your mind is not channeled into a narrow understanding of qi, which would limit your future understanding and development.

A Narrow Definition of Qi 氣之狹義

Now that you understand the general definition of qi, let us look at how qi is defined in qigong society today. As mentioned before, among the three powers, the Chinese have been most concerned with the qi that affects our health and longevity. After four thousand years of emphasizing human qi, when people mention qi, they usually mean the qi circulating in our bodies.

If we look at the Chinese medical and qigong documents that were written in ancient times, the word *qi* was written "炁." This character is constructed of two words: "旡" on the top, which means "nothing," and "灬" on the bottom, which means "fire." This means that the word *qi* was actually written as "no fire" in ancient times. If we go back through Chinese medical and qigong history, it is not hard to understand this expression.

In ancient times, Chinese physicians or qigong practitioners were actually looking for the yin-yang balance of the qi that was circulating in the body. When this goal was reached, there was "no fire" in the internal organs. This concept is very simple. According to Chinese medicine, each of our internal organs needs to receive a specific amount of qi to function properly. If an organ receives an improper amount of qi, usually too much—in other words, too yang or on fire—it will start to malfunction, and in time, physical damage will occur. Therefore, the goal of the medical or qigong practitioners was to attain a state of "no fire," which eventually became the word *qi*.

However, in more recent publications, the qi of "no fire" has been replaced by the word "氣," which is again constructed of two words: "气," which means "air," and "米," which means "rice." This shows that later practitioners realized that after each of us is born, the qi circulating in our bodies is produced mainly by the inhalation of air (oxygen) and the consumption of food (rice). Air is called kong qi (空氣), which literally means "space energy."

For a long time, people were confused about just what type of energy was circulating in our bodies. Many people believed that it was heat, others considered it to be electricity, and still others assumed that it was a mixture of heat, electricity, and light.

This confusion lasted until the early 1980s, when the concept of qi gradually became clear. If we think carefully about what we know from science today, we can see that (except possibly for gravity) there is actually only one type of energy in this universe, and that is electromagnetic energy (electromagnetic waves). This means that light and heat (infrared waves) are also defined as electromagnetic energy. This makes it very clear that the qi circulating in our bodies is actually "bioelectricity," and that our body is a "living electromagnetic field."[1] This field is affected by our thoughts, feelings, activities, the food we eat, the quality of the air we breathe, our lifestyle, the natural energy that surrounds us, and the unnatural energy that modern science inflicts upon us.

2. Traditional Definition of Qigong

Now that you have a clear concept of qi, let us discuss how qigong is traditionally defined. Again, we can define it from a general and a narrow point of view.

A General Definition of Qigong 氣功之廣義

We have explained that qi is energy, and that it is found in heaven, on earth, and in every living thing. In China, the word *gong* (功) is often used instead of *gongfu* (or kung fu, 功夫), which means energy and time. Any study or training that requires a lot of energy and time to learn or to accomplish is called gongfu. The term can be applied to any special skill or study as long as it requires time, energy, and patience. Therefore, the correct definition of qigong is any training or study dealing with qi that takes a long time and a lot of effort. You can see from this definition that qigong is a science that studies the energy in nature. The main difference between this energy science and Western energy science is that qigong focuses on the inner energy of human beings, while Western energy science pays more attention to the energy outside of the human body. When you study

1. *Life's Invisible Current*, by Albert L. Huebner, *East West Journal*, June 1986.

qigong, it is worthwhile to also consider the modern, scientific point of view and not restrict yourself to only the traditional beliefs.

The Chinese have studied qi for thousands of years. Some of the information on the patterns and cycles of nature has been recorded in books, one of which is the *Yi Jing* (易經) (*Book of Changes*; 1122 BCE). When the *Yi Jing* was written, the Chinese people, as mentioned earlier, believed that natural power included heaven (tian, 天), earth (di, 地), and man (ren, 人). These are called the three powers (san cai, 三才) and are manifested by the three qi: heaven qi, earth qi, and human qi. These three facets of nature have their definite rules and cycles. The rules never change, and the cycles are repeated regularly. The Chinese people used an understanding of these natural principles and the *Yi Jing* to calculate the changes of natural qi. This calculation is called the eight trigrams (bagua, 八卦). From the eight trigrams the sixty-four hexagrams are derived. Therefore, the *Yi Jing* was probably the first book that taught the Chinese people about qi and its variations in nature and man. The relationship of the three natural powers and their qi variations were later discussed extensively in the book *Theory of Qi's Variation* (*Qi Hua Lun*, 氣化論).

Understanding heaven qi is very difficult, and it was especially so in ancient times when science was just developing. But because nature is always repeating itself, the experiences accumulated over the years have made it possible to trace the natural patterns. Understanding the rules and cycles of heavenly timing (tian shi, 天時) will help you to understand natural changes of the seasons, climate, weather, rain, snow, drought, and all other natural occurrences. If you observe carefully, you can see many of these routine patterns and cycles caused by the rebalancing of the qi fields. Among the natural cycles are those that repeat every day, month, or year, as well as cycles of twelve years and sixty years.

Earth qi is a part of heaven qi. If you can understand the rules and the structure of the earth, you can understand how mountains and rivers are formed, how plants grow, how rivers move, what part of the country is best for someone, where to build a house and which direction it should face so that it is a healthy place to live, and many other things related to the earth. In China there are people called geomancy teachers (di li shi, 地理師) or wind water teachers (feng shui shi, 風水師), who make their living this way. The term *wind water* (feng shui, 風水) is commonly used because the location and character of the wind and water in a landscape are the most important factors in evaluating a location. These experts use the accumulated body of geomantic knowledge and the *Yi Jing* to help people make important decisions such as where and how to build a house, where to bury their dead, and how to rearrange or redecorate homes and offices so that they are better places to live and work in. Many people even believe that setting up a store or business according to the guidance of feng shui can make it more prosperous.

Among the three qi, human qi is probably the one studied most thoroughly. The study of human qi covers a large number of different subjects. The Chinese people believe that human qi is affected and controlled by heaven qi and earth qi and that they in fact determine your destiny. Therefore, if you understand the relationship between nature and people, in addition to understanding human relations (ren shi, 人事), you can predict wars, the destiny of a country, a person's desires and temperament, and even his future. People who practice this profession are called calculate life teachers (suan ming shi, 算命師).

However, the greatest achievement in the study of human qi is in regard to health and longevity. Because qi is the source of life, if you understand how qi functions and know how to regulate it correctly, you should be able to live a long and healthy life. Remember that you are part of nature, and you are channeled into the cycles of nature. If you go against this natural cycle, you may become sick, so it is in your best interest to follow the way of nature. This is the meaning of "Dao" (道), which can be translated as the "natural way."

Many different aspects of human qi have been researched, including acupuncture, acupressure, massage, herbal treatment, meditation, and qigong exercises. The use of acupuncture, acupressure, and herbal treatment to adjust human qi flow has become the root of Chinese medical science. Meditation and moving qigong exercises are widely used by the Chinese people to improve their health or even to cure certain illnesses. In addition, Daoists and Buddhists use meditation and qigong exercises in their pursuit of enlightenment.

In conclusion, the study of any of the aspects of qi including heaven qi, earth qi, and human qi should be called qigong. However, because the term is usually used today only in reference to the cultivation of human qi through meditation and exercise, we will use it in only this narrower sense to avoid confusion.

A Narrow Definition of Qigong 氣功之狹義

As mentioned earlier, the narrow definition of qi is the "energy circulating in the human body." Therefore, the narrow definition of qigong is the "study or the practice of circulating the qi in the human body." Because our bodies are part of nature, the narrow definition of qigong should also include the study of how our bodies relate to heaven qi and earth qi. Today, Chinese qigong consists of several different fields: acupuncture, herbal treatment, martial arts qigong, qigong massage, qigong exercises, qigong healing, and religious enlightenment qigong. Naturally, these fields are mutually related and in many cases cannot be separated.

In ancient times, qigong was also commonly called tu-na (吐納). Tu-na means to "utter and admit," which implies uttering and admitting the air through the nose. The reason for this is simply that qigong practice is closely related to the methods of how to inhale and exhale correctly. Zhuang Zi (莊子), during the Chinese Warring States Period (403–222 BCE) (戰國) said, "Blowing puffing to breathe, uttering the old and admitting the new, the bear's natural [action] and the bird's extending [the neck], are all for longevity. This is also favored by those people living as long as Peng, Zu [彭祖] who practice dao-yin [i.e., direct-lead, 導引], and nourishing the shapes [i.e., cultivating the physical body]."[2] Peng, Zu was a legendary qigong practitioner during the period of Emperor Yao (堯) (2356–2255 BCE) who was said to have lived for eight hundred years. From this saying, we can see that qigong was also commonly called dao-yin (i.e., direct-lead, 導引), which means to use the mind and physical movements to direct and to lead the qi's circulation in the correct way. The physical movements commonly imitate the natural instinctive movements of animals such as bears and birds. A famous medical qigong set passed down at this time was the Five Animal Sports (Wu Qin Xi, 五禽戲), which imitates the movements of the tiger, deer, bear, ape, and bird.

The Chinese have discovered that the human body has twelve major qi channels (shi er jing, 十二經) (meridians) that branch out with countless secondary channels (luo, 絡). This is similar to the blood circulatory system in the body. The primary channels are like arteries and veins while the secondary channels are like capillaries. The twelve primary channels are like **rivers,** and the secondary channels are like **streams** branching out from the rivers. From this network, the qi is distributed throughout the entire body, connecting the extremities (fingers and toes) to the internal organs and also the skin to the bone marrow. Here you should understand that the internal organs of Chinese medicine do not necessarily correspond to the physical organs as understood in the West, but rather to a set of clinical functions similar to each other and related to the organ system.

The human body also has eight vessels (ba mai, 八脈). The eight vessels, which are often referred to as the extraordinary vessels, function like **reservoirs** and regulate the distribution and circulation of qi in your body. The famous Chinese Daoist medical doctor, Li, Shi-Zhen (李時珍) in his book, *The Study of Strange Meridians and Eight Vessels* (*Qi Jing Ba Mai Kao*, 奇經八脈考) said, "It is because the regular meridians [i.e., twelve primary qi channels] are like rivers, while the strange meridians [i.e., eight vessels] are like lakes. [When] the regular meridians' [qi] is abundant and flourishing, then overflow to the strange meridians."[3] We will discuss the qi network more in the next section of this chapter.

When the qi in the eight reservoirs is full and strong, the qi in the rivers is strong and will be regulated efficiently. When there is stagnation in any of these twelve channels or rivers, the qi that flows to the body's extremities and to the internal organs will be abnormal, and illness may develop. You should understand that every channel has its particular qi flow strength, and every channel is different. All of these different levels of qi strength are affected by your mind, the weather, the time of day, the food you have eaten, and even your mood. For example, when the weather is dry, the qi in the lungs will tend to be more positive (i.e., yang, 陽) than when it is moist. When you are angry, the qi flow in your

2.《莊子刻意》：“吹呴呼吸，吐故納新，熊經鳥伸，為壽而已矣。此導引之士，養形之人，彭祖壽考者之所好也。”

3. 李時珍《奇經八脈考》：“蓋正經猶夫溝渠，奇經猶夫湖澤，正經之脈隆盛，則溢于奇經。”

liver channel will be abnormal. The qi strength in the different channels varies throughout the day in a regular cycle, and at any particular time, one channel is strongest. For example, between 11:00 a.m. and 1:00 p.m., the qi flow in the heart channel is the strongest. Furthermore, the qi level of the same organ can be different from one person to another.

Whenever the qi flow in the twelve rivers or channels is not normal, the eight reservoirs will regulate the qi flow and bring it back into balance. For example, when you experience a sudden shock, the qi flow in the bladder immediately becomes deficient. Normally, the reservoir will immediately regulate the qi in this channel so that you recover from the shock. However, if the reservoir qi is also deficient, or if the effect of the shock is too great and there is not enough time to regulate the qi, the bladder will suddenly contract, causing unavoidable urination.

When a person is sick, his qi level tends to be either too positive (excessive, yang, 陽) or too negative (deficient, yin, 陰). A Chinese physician would either use a prescription of herbs to adjust the qi, or else he would insert acupuncture needles at various spots on the channels to inhibit the flow in some channels and stimulate the flow in others, so that balance could be restored. However, there is another alternative, which is to use certain physical and mental exercises to adjust the qi. In other words, to use qigong exercises.

However, when qigong is defined in scholarly society, it is somewhat different. The qigong practice is focused on regulating the disturbed emotional mind. When the emotional mind is regulated into a peaceful and calm state, the body will be relaxed, which will assist the qi to circulate smoothly in the body and therefore regulate itself into a more harmonious state. From this, mental and physical health can be achieved.

When qigong is defined in Daoist and Buddhist society, it refers to the method or training of leading the qi from the lower dan tian (i.e., elixir field, 下丹田) to the brain for spiritual enlightenment or Buddhahood. The lower dan tian is the place in the abdominal area where one is able to store the qi. It is considered a qi storage area or bioelectric battery. Naturally, its training theory and methods will not be easy. In fact, religious qigong is considered one of the highest levels of qigong training in China.

Finally, when qigong is defined in martial arts society, it refers to the theory and methods of using qi to energize the physical body to its maximum efficiency for manifestation of power. However, because a great portion of martial arts qigong was derived from religious qigong, *Muscle/Tendon Changing and Marrow/Brain Washing Qigong* (*Yi Jin Jing and Xi Sui Jing*, 易筋經、洗髓經), it is not surprising that the profound level of training of martial arts qigong remains the same as that of religious qigong.

To make the above concepts clearer, we will discuss further the different qigong categories later. If you wish to know more about medical qigong, please refer to the books *Qigong for Health & Martial Arts* and *The Root of Chinese Qigong*. If you wish to know more about religious qigong, please refer to the book *Qigong—The Secret of Youth*. If you are interested in martial qigong, the book *The Essence of Shaolin White Crane* is highly recommended. Please see the YMAA website (www.ymaa.com) for more information about these books.

3. Scope of Qigong Practice

Often, people ask me the same question: Is jogging, weight lifting, dancing, or even walking a kind of qigong practice? To answer this question, let us trace back qigong history to before the Chinese Qin and Han dynastic periods (秦、漢，255 BCE–220 CE). Then you can see that the origin of many qigong practices is actually in dancing. Through dancing, the physical body was exercised, and the healthy condition of the physical body was maintained. Also, through dancing and matching movements with music, the mind was regulated into a harmonious state. From this harmonious mind, the spirit was raised to a more energized state or calmed down to a peaceful level. This qigong dancing was later passed to Japan during the Chinese Han dynasty (206 BCE–220 CE) (漢朝) and became a very elegant, slow, and high class of dancing in the Japanese royal court. This taijiquan-like dancing is still practiced in Japan today.

The ways of African or Native American dancing in which the body is bounced up and down also assists in loosening up the joints and improving qi circulation. Naturally, jogging, weight lifting, and even walking are kinds of qigong practices. Therefore, we can say that any activity that is able to regulate the qi circulation in the body is a qigong practice. This can also include the food we eat, the air we breathe, and even emotions and thoughts.

Let us define it more clearly. If laid out in a linear graph with the left vertical line representing the amount of usage of the physical body (yang) and the right vertical line representing the usage of the mind (yin), we can see that the more you practice toward the left, the more physical effort and the less mind are needed. This can be applied to aerobic dancing, walking, or jogging in which the mind usage is relatively small compared to physical action. In this kind of qigong practice, normally you do not need special training, and it is classified as layman qigong. In the middle area, the mind and the physical activity are almost equally important. This kind of qigong will be the slow-moving qigong commonly practiced, in which the mind is used to lead the qi in coordination with the movements. Theoretically speaking, when the body is in its state of slow and relaxed movements, the qi led by the mind can reach the deeper places of the body such as ligaments, marrow, and internal organs. Consequently, the self-internal feeling can also be deep and the qi can be led there significantly. For example, taiji qigong, white crane qigong, snake qigong, dragon qigong, and many others are very typical body-mind qigong exercises. These are specifically practiced in Chinese medical and martial arts societies.

However, when you reach a profound level of qigong practice, the mind becomes more critical. When you reach this high level, you are dealing with your mind while you are sitting or standing still and are extremely relaxed. Most of this level of mental qigong

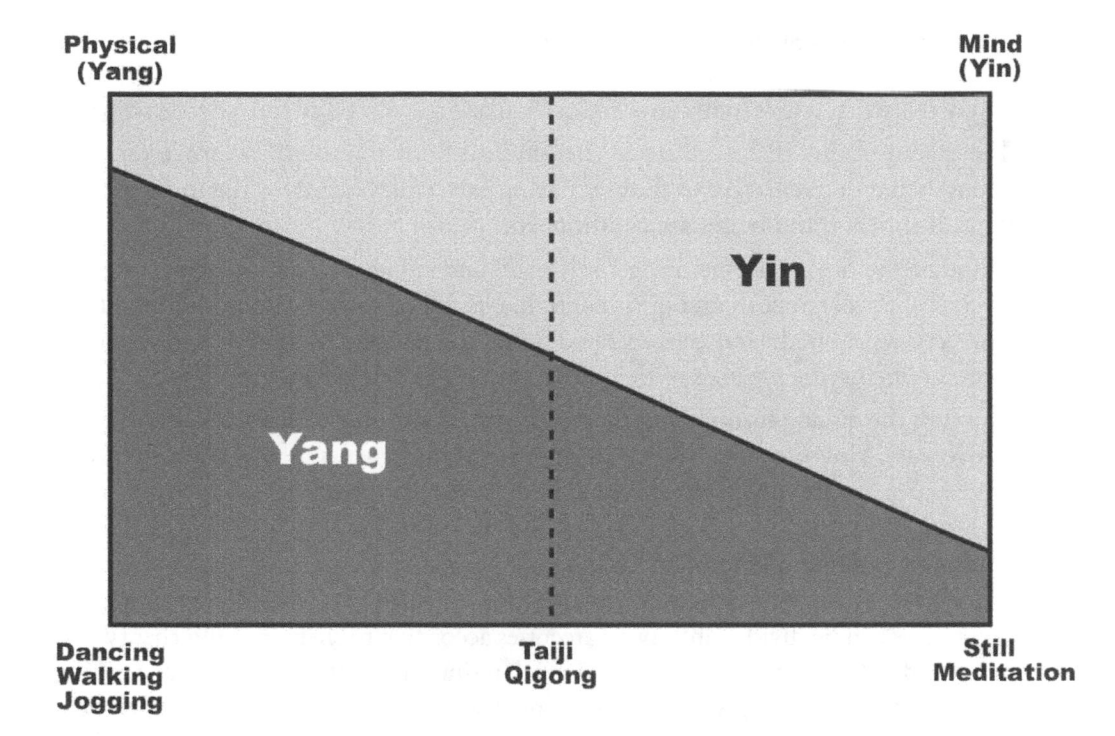

Physical (Yang)

Mind (Yin)

Yin

Yang

Dancing Walking Jogging

Taiji Qigong

Still Meditation

training was practiced by scholars and religious qigong practitioners. In this practice, you may have a little physical movement in the lower abdomen area. However, the main focus of this qigong practice is to cultivate the peaceful and neutral mind and further pursue the final goal of spiritual enlightenment. This kind of qigong practice includes embryonic breathing meditation (taixi jing zuo, 胎息静坐), sitting chan (ren) (坐禪，忍), small circulation meditation (xiao zhou tian, 小周天), grand circulation meditation (da zhou tian, 大周天), or brain washing enlightenment meditation (xi sui gong, 洗髓功).

From this you can see that different qigong practices have different goals. Theoretically speaking, in order to have a good healthy, long, and happy life, both your physical body and your mind must be healthy. The best qigong for health is actually located in the middle of our model, where you learn how to regulate your physical body and also your mind. Naturally, you may practice the yin side through still meditation and the yang side from physical action separately. From this yin and yang balancing practice, your qi can be built up to a more abundant level, and the qi can also be circulated smoothly in the body.

From this, we can conclude the following:

1. Any activity that is able to improve the qi circulation in our body can be called qigong.

2. The qigong forms that emphasize the physical body more will improve physical strength and qi circulation of the areas being exercised. Normally, the muscles, tendons, ligaments, and bones are conditioned.

3. Through the qigong forms using both body and mind, one can achieve a deeper level of physical strength and qi circulation. Normally, with the coordination of the relaxed physical body and concentrated mind, the qi circulation is able to reach the internal organs, deep places of the joints, and even the marrow.

4. Through the qigong forms using mostly the mind, one may reach a profound meditative state. However, due to the lack of physical movements, physical strength will tend to degenerate, unless the physical body is also exercised.

4. Definition of External and Internal Elixirs

Let us now review the traditional classifications of qigong. Generally speaking, all qigong practices can be divided into two categories according to their training theory and methods: wai dan (external elixir, 外丹) and nei dan (internal elixir, 內丹). Understanding the differences between them will give you an overview of most Chinese qigong practice.

Wai Dan (External Elixir) 外丹

Wai (外) means "external" or "outside," and dan (丹) means "elixir." External here means the skin surface of the body or the limbs, as opposed to the torso or the center of the body, which includes all of the vital organs. Elixir is a hypothetical, life-prolonging substance for which Chinese Daoists have been searching for several millennia. They originally thought that the elixir was something physical that could be prepared from herbs or chemicals purified in a furnace. After thousands of years of study and experimentation, they found that the elixir is in the body. In other words, if you want to prolong your life, you must find the elixir in your body and then learn to cultivate, protect, and nourish it. Actually, the elixir is the essence of the inner energy or qi circulating in the body.

There are many ways of producing elixir or qi in the body. In wai dan qigong practice, you may exercise your limbs through dancing or even walking. As you exercise, the qi builds up in your arms and legs. When the qi potential in your limbs builds to a high enough level, the qi will flow through the twelve primary qi channels, clearing any obstructions and flowing into the center of the body to nourish the organs. This is the main reason that a person who works out or has a physical job is generally healthier than someone who sits around all day.

Naturally, you may simply massage your body to produce the qi. Through massage, you may stimulate the cells of your body to a higher energized state, and therefore the qi concentration will be raised and the circulation enhanced. After massage, when you relax, the higher levels of qi on the skin surface and muscles will flow into the center of the body and thereby improve the qi circulatory conditions in your internal organs. This is the theoretical foundation of the tui na (推拿) (i.e., pushing and grabbing) qigong massage.

Through acupuncture, you may also bring the qi level near the skin surface to a higher level, and from this stimulation, the qi condition of the internal organs can be regulated through qi channels. Therefore, acupuncture (dian xue, 點穴) (i.e., cavity press) can also be classified as wai dan qigong practice. Naturally, the herbal treatments are a way of wai dan practice as well.

From this, we can briefly conclude that any possible stimulation or exercise that accumulates a high level of qi in the limbs or at the surface of the body and then flows inward toward the center of the body can be classified as wai dan (external elixir) (Figure 3-2).

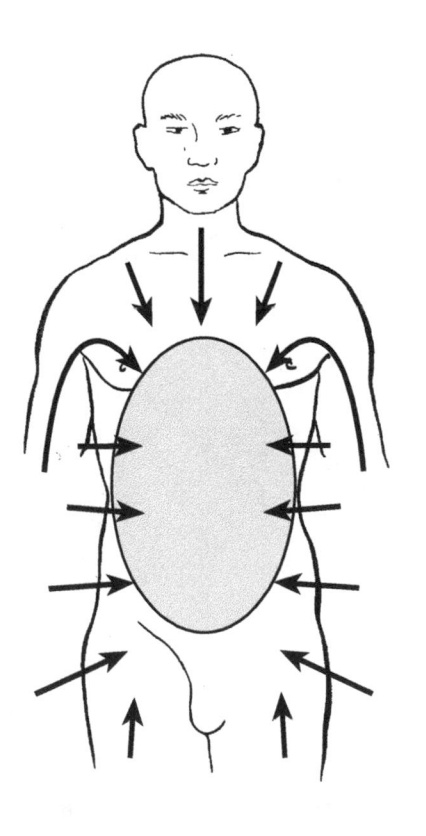

Direction of qi flow during/after external elixir qigong.

Nei Dan (Internal Elixir) 內丹

Nei (內) means "internal" and dan (丹) again means "elixir." Thus, nei dan means to build the elixir internally. Here, internally means inside the body instead of in the limbs.

Normally, the qi is accumulated in the qi vessels instead of the primary qi channels. Whereas in wai dan the qi is built up in the limbs or skin surface and then moved into the body through primary qi channels, nei dan exercises build up qi in the body and lead it out to the limbs. Normally, nei dan qigong is accomplished by special breathing techniques during the meditation process. The first step of nei dan practice is to build up abundant qi in the lower dan tian (i.e., human bioelectric battery). This abundant qi can then be distributed to the eight vessels to increase the store of qi. Only then can the qi circulating in the twelve primary qi channels be regulated smoothly and efficiently.

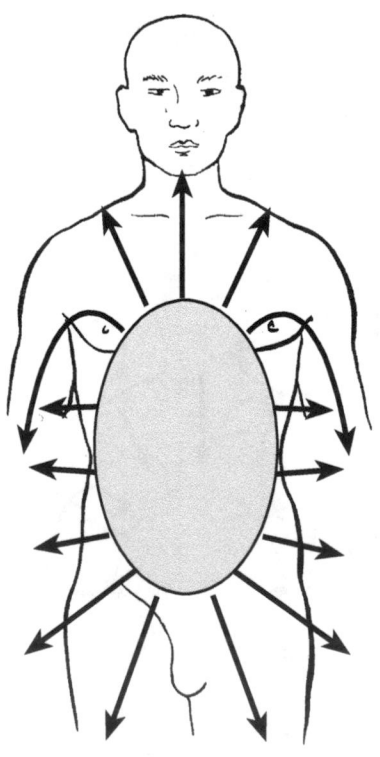

Direction of qi flow during/after internal elixir qigong.

To build up the qi and store it internally, you must first have a profound feeling that allows your mind to reach the deep places of your body. You should know that feeling is the language by which your mind and body communicate. Therefore, to improve the communication ability, your feeling of your physical body and qi body must reach a high level. The training to increase this sensitivity of feeling is called nei shi gongfu (內視功夫), which means the "gongfu of internal vision or observation." In fact, to see or to observe inside your body means to feel it. It is called gongfu (功夫) simply because it will take a great deal of time and practice to reach a high level of accurate feeling.

Generally speaking, nei dan theory is deeper than wai dan theory and is more difficult to understand and practice. Traditionally, most of the nei dan qigong practices have been passed down more secretly than those of the wai dan. This is especially true for the highest levels of nei dan training, such as marrow/brain washing, which were passed down to only a few trusted disciples.

Normally, the first step of practicing internal elixir qigong has been known by Daoists as small cyclic heaven (xiao zhou tian, 小周天) or small circulation meditation. This is also commonly known as microcosmic meditation in yoga (yujia, 瑜珈) or as turning the wheel of natural law (zhuan fa lun, 轉法輪) by Buddhist society.

Small circulation can be considered as the foundation of the internal elixir qigong. Through practicing small circulation meditation, a practitioner can circulate the qi (bioelectricity) smoothly in the conception and governing vessels (ren and du mai, 任‧督脈), the two major qi vessels that regulate the qi circulating in the twelve primary qi channels (shi er jing, 十二經). After completing small circulation, a practitioner will learn grand cyclic heaven (da zhou tian, 大周天) or grand circulation. This is also commonly called macrocosmic meditation in Indian yoga. Through grand circulation meditation practice, a practitioner will learn how to circulate the qi throughout his body and then learn to exchange the qi with partners or surrounding environments. The purpose of grand circulation meditation is to reopen the heaven eye (tian yan, 天眼) (i.e., the third eye) so as to unify the natural spirit and human spirit (tian ren he yi, 天人合一). This is the ultimate goal of spiritual enlightenment in both Daoism and Buddhism.

To reach the goal of internal elixir qigong practice, a practitioner must first know how to store the qi to an abundant level in the real lower dan tian (zhen xia dan tian, 真下丹田) (i.e., human biobattery) using the theory and the techniques of embryonic breathing (tai xi, 胎息). These were kept top secret in ancient qigong society. It was not until the second half of the last century that documents expounding on embryonic breathing were gradually revealed to the general public. If you are interested in studying embryonic breathing, please refer to my book *Qigong Meditation—Embryonic Breathing*, by YMAA Publication Center.

5. Schools of Qigong Practice

We can also classify qigong into four major categories according to the purpose or final goal of the training: (A) curing sickness, (B) maintaining health, (C) enlightenment or Buddhahood, and (D) martial arts. These are only general guidelines, however, because almost every style of qigong serves more than one of the above purposes. For example, although martial qigong focuses on increasing fighting effectiveness, it can also improve your health. Daoist qigong aims for longevity and enlightenment, but to reach this goal, you need to be in good health and know how to cure sickness. Because of this multipurpose aspect of the categories, it will be simpler to discuss their backgrounds rather than the goals of their training. Knowing the history and basic principles of each category will help you to understand their qigong more clearly.

Medical Qigong—For Healing

In ancient Chinese society, most emperors respected the scholars and were affected by their philosophy. Doctors were not regarded highly because they made their diagnosis by touching the patient's body, which was considered characteristic of the lower classes in society. Although doctors developed a profound and successful medical science, they were commonly looked down on by society. However, they continued to work hard and study, and they quietly passed down the results of their research to succeeding generations.

Of all the groups studying qigong in China, doctors pursued it the longest. Since the discovery of qi circulation in the human body about four thousand years ago, Chinese doctors have devoted a major portion of their efforts to studying the behavior of qi. Their efforts resulted in acupuncture, acupressure or cavity press massage, and herbal treatment.

In addition, many Chinese doctors used their medical knowledge to create different sets of qigong exercises either for maintaining health or for curing specific illnesses. Chinese medical doctors believed that doing only sitting or still meditation to regulate the body, mind, and breathing, as the scholars qigong or Buddhist Chan (禪) (i.e., Zen, 忍) meditation did, was not enough to cure sickness. They believed that in order to increase the qi circulation, you must move. Although a calm and peaceful mind was important for health, exercising the body was more important. They learned through their medical practice that people who exercised properly were sick less often, and their bodies degenerated less quickly than was the case with people who just sat around. They also realized that specific body movements could increase the qi circulation in specific organs. They reasoned from this that these exercises could also be used to treat specific illnesses and to restore the normal functioning of the organs.

Some of these movements are similar to the way in which certain animals move. For an animal to survive in the wild, it must instinctively know how to protect its body. Part of this instinct is concerned with how to build up its qi, and how to keep its qi from being lost. We humans have lost many of these instincts over the years that we have been separating ourselves from nature.

Many doctors developed qigong exercises that were modeled after animal movements to maintain health and cure sickness. A typical, well-known set of such exercises is wu qin xi (五禽戲) (five animal sports) created by Dr. Hua Tuo (華佗) nearly two thousand years ago. (Others say wu qin xi was created by Jun Qing [君倩] and was publicized by Hua Tuo.) Another famous set based on similar principles is called ba duan jin (八段錦) (eight pieces of brocade). It was created by Marshal Yue, Fei (岳飛) during Chinese Southern Song dynasty (南宋) (1127–1280 CE). Yue, interestingly enough, was a soldier and scholar rather than a doctor.

In addition, using their medical knowledge of qi circulation, Chinese doctors researched until they found which movements could help cure particular illnesses and health problems. Not surprisingly, many of these movements were not unlike the ones used to maintain health because many illnesses are caused by unbalanced qi. When an imbalance continues for a long time, the organs will be affected and may be physically damaged. It is just like running a machine without supplying the proper electrical current; over time, the machine will be damaged. Chinese doctors believe that before physical damage to an organ shows up in a patient's body, there is first an abnormality in the qi balance and circulation. Abnormal qi circulation is the very beginning of illness and organ damage. When qi is too positive (yang) or too negative (yin) in a specific organ's qi channel, your physical organ begins to suffer damage. If you do not correct the qi circulation, that organ will malfunction or degenerate. The best way to heal someone is to adjust and balance the qi even before there is any physical problem. Therefore, correcting or increasing the normal qi circulation is the major goal of acupuncture or acupressure treatments. Herbs and special diets are also considered important treatments in regulating the qi in the body.

As long as the illness is limited to the level of qi stagnation and there is no physical organ damage, the qigong exercises used for maintaining health can be used to readjust the qi circulation and treat the problem. However, if the sickness is already so serious that the physical organs have started to fail, then the situation has become critical and a specific treatment is necessary. The treatment can include acupuncture, herbs, or even an operation, as well as specific qigong exercises designed to accelerate healing. For example, ulcers and asthma can often be cured or helped by some simple exercises. Recently in both mainland China and Taiwan, certain qigong exercises have been shown to be effective in treating certain kinds of cancer.

Over thousands of years of observing nature and themselves, some qigong practitioners went even deeper. They realized that the body's qi circulation changes with the seasons and that it is a good idea to help the body out during these periodic adjustments. They also noticed that in each season, different organs have characteristic problems. For example, in the beginning of autumn, the lungs must adapt to the colder air that you are breathing. While this adjustment is going on, the lungs are susceptible to disturbance, so your lungs may feel uncomfortable, and you may easily catch colds. Your digestive system is also affected during seasonal changes. Your appetite may increase, or you may have diarrhea. When your temperature drops, your kidneys and bladder will start to give you trouble. For example, if the kidneys are stressed, you may feel pain in the back. Focusing on these seasonal qi disorders, the meditators created a set of movements that can be used to speed up the body's adjustment.

In addition to Marshal Yue, Fei, many people who were not doctors also created sets of medical qigong. These sets were probably originally created to maintain health and were also later used for curing sickness.

Scholar Qigong—For Maintaining Health

In China before the Han dynasty, there were two major schools of scholarship. One of them was created by Confucius (孔子) (551–479 BCE) during the Spring and Autumn

Period (Chun Qiu, 春秋) (722–484 BCE). Later, his philosophy was popularized and expanded by Mencius (孟子) (372–289 BCE) in the Warring States Period (Zhan Guo, 戰國) (403–222 BCE). The scholars who practice his philosophy are commonly called Confucians or Confucianists (Ru Jia, 儒家). The key words to their basic philosophy are loyalty (zhong, 忠), filial piety (xiao, 孝), humanity (ren, 仁), kindness (ai, 愛), trust (xin, 信), justice (yi, 義), harmony (he, 和), and peace (ping, 平). Humanity and human feelings are the main subjects of study. Confucius's philosophy has become the center of much of Chinese culture.

The second major school of scholarship was called Daoism (Dao Jia, 道家) and was created by Lao Zi (老子) (604–531 BCE). Lao Zi is considered to be the author of the book the *Dao De Jing* (*Classic on the Virtue of the Dao*) (道德經), which describes the "virtue of the Dao such as human moralities." Later, in the Warring States Period, his follower Zhuang Zhou (莊周) wrote a book called *Zhuang Zi* (莊子), which led to the formation of another strong branch of Daoism. Before the Han dynasty, Daoism was considered a branch of scholarship. However, in the Eastern Han dynasty (25–168 CE), traditional Daoism was combined with the Buddhism imported from India by Zhang, Dao-Ling (張道陵); it gradually began to be treated as a religion. Therefore, the Daoism before the Han dynasty should be considered scholarly Daoism rather than religious.

With regard to their contribution to qigong, both schools emphasized maintaining health and preventing disease. They believed that many illnesses are caused by mental and emotional excesses. When a person's mind is not calm, balanced, and peaceful, the organs will not function normally. For example, depression can cause stomach ulcers and indigestion. Anger will cause the liver to malfunction. Sadness will cause stagnation and tightness in the lungs. Fear can disturb the normal functioning of the kidneys and bladder. They realized that if you want to avoid illness, you must learn to balance and relax your thoughts and emotions. This is called regulating the mind (tiao xin, 調心).

Therefore, scholars emphasized gaining a peaceful mind through meditation. In their still meditation, the main part of the training is getting rid of thoughts so that the mind is clear and calm. When you become calm, the flow of thoughts and emotions slows down, and you feel mentally and emotionally neutral. This kind of meditation can be thought of as practicing emotional self-control. When you are in this "no thought" state, you become very relaxed and can even relax deep down into your internal organs. When your body is this relaxed, your qi will naturally flow smoothly and strongly. This kind of still meditation was very common in ancient Chinese scholar society.

To reach the goal of a calm and peaceful mind, their training focused on regulating the mind, body, and breath. They believed that as long as these three things were regulated, the qi flow would be smooth, and sickness would not occur. This is why the qi training of the scholars is called xiu qi (修氣), which means "cultivating qi." Xiu (修) in Chinese means to regulate, to cultivate, to repair, or to maintain in good condition. This is very different from the religious Daoist qi training after the Eastern Han dynasty. It was called lian qi (練氣) and is translated as "train qi." Lian (練) means to drill or to practice to make stronger. They believed that it is possible to train your qi to make it stronger and to extend your life. It is said in scholarly society, "In human life, seventy is rare."[4] You should understand that few of the common people in ancient times lived past seventy because of the lack of good food and modern medical technology. It is also said, "peace with heaven and delight in your destiny" (安天樂命) and "cultivate the body and await destiny" (修身俟命). Compare this with the philosophy of the later Daoists, who said, "one hundred and twenty means dying young."[5] They believed and have proven that human life can be lengthened, and destiny can be resisted and overcome.

Confucianism and Daoism were the two major scholarly schools in China, but there were many other schools that were also more or less involved in qigong practices. We will not discuss them here because there are only a very limited number of qigong documents from these other schools.

Religious Qigong—For Enlightenment or Buddhahood

Religious qigong, though not as popular as other categories in China, is recognized as having achieved the highest accomplishments of all the qigong categories. It used to be kept secret in monastic society, and only in the twentieth century was it revealed to laymen.

In China, religious qigong includes mainly Daoist and Buddhist qigong. The main purpose of their training is striving for enlightenment (shen tong, 神通), or what the Buddhists refer to as Buddhahood (cheng fo, 成佛). They are looking for a way to lift themselves above normal human suffering and to escape from the cycle of continual reincarnation. They believe that all human suffering is caused by the seven passions and six desires (qi qing liu yu, 七情六慾). The seven passions are happiness (xi, 喜), anger (nu, 怒), sorrow (ai, 哀), joy (le, 樂), love (ai, 愛), hate (hen, 恨), and desire (yu, 慾). The six desires are the six sensory pleasures derived from the eyes, ears, nose, tongue, body, and mind. If you are still bound to these emotions and desires, you will reincarnate after your death. To avoid reincarnation, you must train your spirit to reach a very high stage where it is strong enough to be independent after your death. This spirit will enter the heavenly kingdom and gain eternal peace. This final stage of training is called unification of heaven and man (tian ren he yi, 天人合一). This training is hard to do in the everyday world, so practitioners frequently flee society and move into the solitude of the mountains, where they can concentrate all of their energies on self-cultivation.

Religious qigong practitioners train to strengthen their internal qi to nourish their shen (神) (i.e., spirit) until the shen is able to survive the death of the physical body. Marrow/brain washing qigong (xi sui gong, 洗髓功) training is necessary to reach this

4. "人生七十古來稀。"
5. 一百二十謂之天。

stage. It enables them to lead qi to the brain, where the shen resides, and raise the brain cells to a higher energy state. This training used to be restricted to only a few priests who had reached an advanced level. Tibetan Buddhists were also heavily involved in this training. Over the last two thousand years, Tibetan Buddhists, Chinese Buddhists, and religious Daoists have followed the same principles to become the three major religious schools of qigong training.

This religious striving toward enlightenment or Buddhahood is recognized as the highest and most difficult level of qigong. Many qigong practitioners reject the rigors of this religious striving and practice marrow/brain washing qigong solely for the purpose of longevity. It was these people who eventually revealed the secrets of marrow/brain washing to the outside world. If you are interested in knowing more about this training, you may refer to the author's book *Qigong–The Secret of Youth*, by YMAA Publication Center.

Martial Qigong—For Fighting

Chinese martial qigong was probably not developed until Da Mo (達磨) wrote the *Muscle/Tendon Changing and Marrow/Brain Washing Qigong Classic* (*Yi Jin Jing, Xi Sui Jing*; 易筋經‧洗髓經) in the Shaolin Temple (少林寺) during the Liang dynasty (梁朝) (502–557 CE). When Shaolin monks trained in Da Mo's muscle/tendon changing qigong, they found they could not only improve their health but also greatly increase the power of their martial techniques. Since then, many martial styles have developed qigong sets to increase their fighting effectiveness. In addition, many martial styles have been created based on qigong theory. Martial artists have played a major role in Chinese qigong society.

When qigong theory was first applied to the martial arts, it was used to increase the power and efficiency of the muscles. The theory is very simple: the mind (yi) is used to lead qi to the muscles to energize them so that they function more efficiently. The average person generally uses his muscles at about 40 percent of maximum efficiency. If one can train concentration and use strong yi (意) (i.e., the mind generated from clear thinking) to lead qi to the muscles effectively, one can energize the muscles to a higher level and therefore increase fighting effectiveness.

As acupuncture theory became better understood, fighting techniques were able to reach even more advanced levels. Martial artists learned to attack specific areas, such as vital acupuncture cavities, to disturb the enemies' qi flow and create imbalances that caused injury or even death. To do this, the practitioner must understand the route and timing of the qi circulation in the human body. He also has to train so that he can strike the cavities accurately and to the correct depth. These cavity-strike techniques are called dian xue (點穴) (pointing cavities) or dian mai (點脈) (pointing vessels).

Most of the martial qigong practices help to improve the practitioner's health. However, there are other martial qigong practices that, although they build up some special skill that is useful for fighting, also damage the practitioner's health. An example of this is iron sand palm (tie sha zhang, 鐵砂掌). Although this training can build up amazing destructive power, it can also harm your hands and affect the qi circulation in the hands and internal organs.

Since the sixth century, many martial styles have been created that were based on Da Mo's qigong theory and methods. They can be roughly divided into external and internal styles.

The external styles emphasize building qi in the limbs to coordinate with the physical martial techniques. They follow the theory of wai dan (external elixir) qigong, which usually generates qi in the limbs through special exercises. The concentrated mind is used during the exercises to energize the qi. This significantly increases muscular strength and therefore increases the effectiveness of the martial techniques. Qigong can also be used to train the body to resist punches and kicks. In this training, qi is led to energize the skin and the muscles, enabling them to resist a blow without injury. This training is commonly called iron shirt (tie bu shan, 鐵布衫) or golden bell cover (jin zhong zhao, 金鐘罩). The martial styles that use wai dan qigong training are normally called external styles (wai jia, 外家). Hard qigong training is called hard gong (ying gong, 硬功). Shaolin gongfu is a typical example of a style that uses wai dan martial qigong.

Although wai dan qigong can help the martial artist increase his power, there is a disadvantage. Because wai dan qigong emphasizes training the external muscles, it can cause overdevelopment. This can cause a problem called energy dispersion (san gong, 散功) when the practitioner gets older. To remedy this, when an external martial artist reaches a high level of external qigong training, he will start training internal qigong, which specializes in curing the energy dispersion problem. That is why it is said, "External gongfu is from external to internal."

Internal martial qigong is based on the theory of nei dan (internal elixir). In this method, qi is generated in the body instead of the limbs, and this qi is then led to the limbs to increase power. To lead qi to the limbs, the techniques must be soft, and muscle usage must be kept to a minimum. The training and theory of nei dan martial qigong is much more difficult than those of wai dan martial qigong. Interested readers should refer to the author's book *Tai Chi Chuan Martial Power*, published by YMAA Publication Center.

Several internal martial styles were created in the Wudang (武當山) and Emei (峨嵋山) Mountains. Popular styles are taijiquan (太極拳), baguazhang (八卦掌), liu he ba fa (六合八法), and xingyiquan (形意拳). However, you should understand that even the internal martial styles, which are commonly called soft styles (ruan quan, 軟拳), must on some occasions use muscular strength while fighting. To have strong power in the fight, the qi must be led to the muscular body and manifested externally. Therefore, once an internal martial artist has achieved a degree of competence in internal qigong, he or she should also learn how to use harder, more external techniques. That is why it is said, "The internal styles are from internal to external and from soft to hard."

You can see that, although qigong is widely studied in Chinese martial society, the main focus of training was originally on increasing fighting ability rather than health.

Good health was considered a by-product of training. It was not until this century that the health aspect of martial qigong started receiving greater attention. This is especially true in the internal martial arts. If you would like to know more about martial qigong, please refer to the book *The Essence of Shaolin White Crane*, published by YMAA Publication Center.

From the above brief summary, you may obtain a general concept of how Chinese qigong can be categorized and should not have further doubt about any qigong you are training.

6. Theories of Yin-Yang and Kan-Li 陰陽、坎離之理論

To practice qigong accurately, you must not only understand the theory but also the correct methods of practice. Knowing the theory correctly places a clear and accurate map in your hands leading you to your goal in the shortest time. Without this map, you may take many years to find the correct path.

Two of the most important concepts in qigong practice are the theory of yin and yang and of kan and li. These two concepts have been commonly confused in qigong society, even in China. If you are able to understand them clearly, you will have grasped an important key to the practice of qigong.

What Are Kan and Li?

Kan and li training has long been of major importance to qigong practitioners. To understand why, you must understand these two words and the theory behind them. The terms *kan* (坎) and *li* (離) occur frequently in qigong documents. In the eight trigrams, kan represents "water," while li represents "fire." However, the everyday terms for water and fire are also often used.

First you should understand that even though kan-li and yin-yang are related, kan and li are not yin and yang. Kan is water, which is able to cool your body down and make it more yin, while li is fire, which warms your body and makes it more yang. Kan and li are the methods or causes, while yin and yang are the results. When kan and li are correctly adjusted or regulated, yin and yang will be balanced and interact harmoniously.

Qigong practitioners believe that your body is always too yang, unless you are sick or have not eaten for a long time, in which case, your body may be more yin. When your body is always yang, it is degenerating and burning out. It is believed that this is the cause of aging. If you are able to use water to cool down your body, you can slow down the process of degeneration and thereby lengthen your life. This is the main reason why qigong practitioners have been studying ways of improving the quality of water in their bodies and of reducing the quantity of fire. I believe that as a qigong practitioner, you should always keep this subject at the top of your list for study and research. If you earnestly ponder and experiment, you can grasp the trick of adjusting them.

If you want to learn how to adjust them, you must understand that water and fire mean many things in your body. The first concern is your qi. Qi is classified as fire or water. When your qi is not pure and causes your physical body to heat up and your mental/spiritual body to become unstable (yang), it is classified as fire qi. The qi that is pure and is able to cool both your physical and spiritual bodies (make them more yin) is considered water qi. However, your body can never be purely water. Water can cool down the fire, but it must never totally quench it because then you would be dead. It is also said that fire qi is able to agitate and stimulate the emotions and from these emotions generate a "mind." This mind is called xin (心) and is considered the fire mind, yang mind, or emotional mind. On the other hand, the mind that water qi generates is calm, steady, and wise. This mind is called yi (意) and is considered to be the water mind or wisdom mind. If your shen is nourished by fire qi, although your shen may be high, it will be scattered and confused (a yangshen). Naturally, if the shen is nourished and raised by water qi, it will be firm and steady (a yin mind). When your yi is able to effectively govern your emotional xin, your will (strong emotional intention) can be firm.

You can see from this discussion that your qi is the main cause of the yin and yang of your physical body, your mind, and your shen. To regulate your body's yin and yang, you must learn how to regulate your body's water and fire qi, and to do this efficiently you must know their sources.

To understand kan and li clearly and to adjust them efficiently, you are urged to use the modern scientific, medical point of view to analyze the concepts. This will allow you to marry the past and present and give birth to the future.

Kan and Li in Breathing, Mind, and Shen

Here we introduce the general concepts of how kan and li relate to your breathing, mind, and shen. Then we will combine them and construct a secret key that will lead you to the qigong treasure.

A. Breathing's Kan and Li

In qigong, breathing is considered a "strategy" that enables you to lead the qi effectively. For example, you can use your breath to lead the qi to your skin or marrow. Slow or fast breathing can make the flow of qi calm or vigorous. When you are excited your body is yang, and you exhale more than you inhale. This leads the qi to the skin so that you sweat, and the excess dissipates into the surrounding air. When you are sad, your body is yin, and you inhale more than you exhale to lead the qi inward to conserve it, and you feel cold. You can see that breathing can be the main cause of changing the body's yin and yang. Therefore, breathing has kan and li.

Generally speaking, in the normal state of your body, inhaling is considered to be a water activity (kan) because you lead the qi inward to the bone marrow where it is stored. This reduces the qi in the muscles and tendons, which calms down the body's yang. Exhaling is considered a fire activity (li) because it brings qi outward to the muscles, tendons, and skin to energize them, making the body more yang. When the body is more yang than its surroundings, the qi in the body is automatically dissipated outward.

Normally, yin and yang should be balanced so that your body will function harmoniously. The trick to maintaining this balance is using breathing strategy. Usually, your inhalations and exhalations should be equal. However, when you are excited, your body is too yang, so you may inhale longer and deeper to calm your mind and lead the qi inside your body to make it more yin.

In qigong practice, it is very important to grasp the trick of correct breathing. It is the exhalation that leads qi to the five centers (head, two laogong cavities at the center of the palms, and two yongquan cavities near the center of the soles) and the skin to exchange qi with the surroundings. Inhalation leads qi deep inside your body to reach the internal organs and marrow. Table 1-1 summarizes how different breathing strategies affect the body's yin and yang in their various manifestations.

B. The Mind's Kan and Li

According to Chinese tradition, a human has two minds: xin (心) and yi (意). Xin is translated literally as "heart" and is considered as the mind generated from emotional disturbance. Therefore, xin can be translated as "emotional mind." The Chinese word for yi is constructed of three characters. The top one means "establish" (立), the middle one means "speaking" (曰), and the bottom one is "heart" (心). That means the emotional mind is under control when you speak. Therefore, yi can be translated as "wisdom mind" or "rational mind." Because the emotional mind makes you excited and emotionally disturbed, which results in the excitement of your body (yang), it is considered as li. The wisdom mind that makes you calm, peaceful, and able to think clearly (yin) is considered to be kan.

In qigong training, the mind is considered the "general" who directs the entire battle. It is the general who decides the fighting strategy (breathing) and controls the movement of the soldiers (qi). Therefore, as a general, you must control your xin (emotional mind), use your yi (wisdom mind) to judge and understand the situation, and then finally decide on the proper strategy.

In qigong, your wisdom mind must first dominate the situation and generate an idea. This idea generates and executes the strategy (breathing) and is also the force that moves the qi. Generally speaking, when your mind is excited, aggressive, and energized, the strategy (breathing) is more offensive (emphasizing exhalation), and the qi circulation is more vigorous and expansive. This aggressive mind is then considered a fire mind because it is able to make your body more yang. However, when the strategy is more defensive (i.e., emphasizing inhalation), the qi circulation will be more calm and condensing. Therefore, a calm or depressed mind is considered a water mind because it can make your body more yin.

You can see that the kan and li of the mind are more important than those of breathing. After all, it is the mind that makes the strategy. Regulating the mind and the breathing are two of the basic techniques for controlling your body's yin and yang. Regulating the mind and the breathing cannot be separated. When the mind is regulated, the breathing can be regulated. When the breathing is regulated, the mind is able to enter a deeper level of calmness.

C. The Shen's Kan and Li

Now it is time to consider the final and most decisive element in winning a battle: the shen (神). Shen is compared to the morale of the general's officers and soldiers. There are many cases throughout history of armies winning battles against great odds because the morale of their soldiers was high. If a soldier's morale is high enough, he can defeat ten enemies.

It is the same in qigong training. It is the shen that determines how successful your qigong practice will be. Your yi (wisdom mind), which is the general who makes the strategy, must also be concerned with raising the fighting morale (shen) of the soldiers (qi). When their morale is raised, the soldiers can be led more efficiently, and consequently, the strategy can be executed more effectively.

You can see that knowing how to use the yi to raise the shen is the major key to successful qigong training. In qigong, shen is considered the headquarters that governs the qi. As a matter of fact, both yi and shen govern the qi. They are closely related and cannot be separated.

Generally speaking, when the wisdom mind (yi) is energized, the shen is also raised. You should understand that in qigong training, you want to raise your shen but not let it get excited. When the shen is raised, the strategy can be carried out effectively. However, if the shen is excited, the body will become too yang, and that is not desirable in qigong practice. When you are practicing qigong, you want to keep your shen high all the time and use it to govern the strategy and the qi. This will enable you to readjust or regulate your kan and li efficiently.

Shen is the control tower that is able to adjust the kan and li, but it does not have kan and li itself. Nevertheless, some qigong practitioners consider the raised shen to be li (fire) and the calm shen to be kan (water).

Now, let us draw a few important conclusions from the above discussion:

a. Kan (water) and li (fire) are not yin and yang. Kan and li are methods that can cause yin or yang.

b. Qi itself is only a form of energy and does not have kan and li. When qi is too excessive or too deficient, it can cause the body to be too yang or too yin.

c. When you adjust kan and li in the body, the mind is the first concern. The mind can be kan or li. It determines the strategy (breathing) for withdrawing the qi (kan) or expanding it (li).

d. Breathing has kan and li. Usually inhaling, which makes the body more yin, is kan. Exhaling, which makes the body more yang, is li.

e. The shen does not have kan and li. Shen is the key to making the kan and li adjustment effective and efficient.

The Key Secrets of Adjusting Kan and Li

In light of these conclusions, let us discuss the keys of kan and li adjustment. These keys are repeatedly mentioned in the ancient documents. The first key is that shen and breathing mutually rely on each other. The second key is that shen and qi mutually combine and harmonize with each other.

A. Shen and Breathing Mutually Dependent (Shen Xi Xiang Yi, 神息相依)

We know that breathing is the strategy that directs the qi in various ways and therefore controls and adjusts the kan and li, which in turn control the body's yin and yang. We also know that the shen is the control tower that is able to make the strategy work in the most efficient way. Therefore, shen governs the strategy directly and controls kan and li and the body's yin and yang indirectly. You can see that the success of your kan and li adjustment depends upon your shen.

When the shen matches your inhaling and exhaling, it can lead the qi to condense and expand in the most efficient way. Your shen must match with the breathing to be raised or calmed down, and the breathing must rely on the shen to make the strategy work efficiently. In this case, it seems that the shen and breathing are depending on each other and cannot be separated. In qigong practice, this training is called shen xi xiang yi (神息相依), which means "shen and breathing depend on each other." When your shen and breathing are matching each other, it is called shen xi (神息) (i.e., shen breathing) because it seems that your shen is actually doing the breathing.

You can see that shen xi xiang yi is a technique or method in which, when the shen and breathing are united, the shen is able to control the qi more directly.

B. Shen and Qi Mutually Combined (Shen Qi Xiang He, 神氣相合)

When your shen and breathing are able to match with each other as one, then the qi can be led directly, and thus shen and qi become one. In qigong practice it is called shen qi xiang he (神氣相合), which means "shen and qi mutually combined or harmonized." When this happens, the shen can govern the qi directly and more efficiently. You can see from this that the shen and qi combining is the result of the shen and breathing being mutually dependent.

Da Mo (達磨) believed that in order to have a long and peaceful life, shen and qi must be coordinated and harmonized with each other. He said, "If [one] does not know how to keep the mother [qi] and son [shen] together, though the qi [is directed] by breathing internally, [nevertheless] the shen is labored and craves external [objects], resulting in the shen being always debauched and dirty; the shen is thus not clear. [If] the shen is not clear, the original harmonious qi will disperse gradually, [shen and qi] cannot be kept together."[6] From this, you can see that shen is very important. To regulate the shen is one of the highest levels of qigong practice. The reason for this is simply that in order to reach a high level of harmony, you must first regulate your emotional mind. This is hard to achieve in lay society.

3-2. Fundamental Theory

In this section, we will explain the fundamental theory behind the two qigong practices in this book: ground qigong exercises and tui na / acupressure massage. However, first let us review the basic theory of its foundation.

General Basic Theory

1. Hormone productions increase during sleep, and the body's metabolism increases, with cell replacement and multiplication taking place. During this biochemical reaction process, a lot of waste is released and accumulated in the body. The way of getting rid of this waste is through enhancing the blood and qi circulation. The ways of reaching these goals are correct qigong exercises and tui na / acupressure massages. Exercises pump the blood and enhance its circulation, stretching open the joints and tightened physical body. These actions expedite the repelling of waste in the body, especially early morning.

2. Through stretching and correct movements, the weak areas of the body, such as the lower back, can be conditioned. When you exercise gradually and progressively each day, the body can be conditioned over time. Before you know it, you have built up your body to a stronger level. Consistent practice is the key of this success.

3. As mentioned in the previous section, through the twelve primary qi channels (meridians), the qi is distributed to the entire body. One end of each channel connects to the defined twelve organs, and the other end connects to the fingertips or toes. Through correct relaxed body movements and stretching, the body can reach a high level of relaxation. When the body is relaxed, the channels will be wide opened for the circulation of qi; thus, the qi circulation in these twelve channels can be enhanced. Qi is the energy of the body. When qi circulates smoothly and abundantly, the life force is increased, and the health is maintained. Naturally, the blood circulation can also be enhanced.

4. Tui na / acupressure massages stimulate qi channels and cavities. When correct channels and cavities are stimulated, the qi's circulation in the channels can be enhanced. Naturally, health can be maintained.

6.《達摩大師住世留形內真妙用訣》: "若不知子母相守，氣雖呼吸於于內，神常勞役于外，遂使神常穢濁而神不清，神既不清，即元和之氣漸散，而不能相守也。"

Meridian Qigong and Yoga Theory

1. Loosening Up Movements (暖身、鬆身運動)

Warming up is usually the first step before any heavy exercise. When you have the right warm-up exercises, you will have excited the cells to a good level. This will increase the effectiveness of later exercises. For example, if you do warm-up exercises before you run or swim, you loosen the body and prevent the muscles from cramping.

When you warm up your body, move the muscles as little as possible. Use only those muscles required. When you lie down, all the muscles are relaxed. This will provide you a great position to loosen up the body.

In practice, you may first loosen up your limbs so the channels to the extremities are opened. After that, loosen up your torso and neck. Naturally, you may first loosen up your torso and neck and then the legs and arms. In this case, you first bring your torso and neck to higher level of relaxation and then open up the channels on the limbs.

2. When you practice, remember to breathe naturally and smoothly. Don't hold your breath. Holding the breath can tighten your body. Breathe softly, gently, and slenderly.

3. When you loosen up the joints, don't use the muscles/tendons on that specific joint. For example, if you wish to loosen up your wrist, and you use the muscles/tendons on the wrist, it will be tensed. The way to loosen up the wrist is to move the elbow and allow the wrist to move with it automatically.

4. As mentioned earlier, stretching the muscles/tendons especially in the joint areas will open up the channels. In addition, through stretching, the body can be conditioned. When you stretch, you should stretch gradually. If you proceed with your stretching too aggressively, you may tear muscles and ligaments. In addition, you should stretch using different angles so different muscles/tendons and ligaments can be stretched. Naturally, you should not hold your breath as you stretch. When you stretch, you should feel comfortable. Remember, comfortable pain improves qi and blood circulation. Significant pain will only cause tightness and make the circulation stagnate and possibly damage the joint.

5. Correct qigong exercises offer better benefits and results. Usually, it takes a qigong master a lifetime of experience to reach a high level of knowledge in knowing if the exercises are correct and effective. To establish this knowledge, when you practice, you should pay attention to your feeling. Feeling is the language that allows your mind and body to communicate. With deep feeling, you can direct your exercises to deeper areas. For example, when you condition your lower back, you want to reach the ligaments connecting the vertebrae. If your feeling is shallow, then the benefit you gain remains shallow. This inner deep feeling is called gongfu of internal vision (內視功夫) and means "the practice of inner understanding through feeling." It is called gongfu (功夫) because it takes a lot of practice to reach the deep feeling.

6. When you stretch, you should increase the duration of your stretching gradually so the body can be gradually conditioned. If you progress too quickly and aggressively, you may injure yourself. Naturally, how much of each exercise a person should do depends

on each individual. That means you have to give yourself a test and see how much you can handle.

7. Recovery includes both mental and physical. Mental recovery means to bring your mind to a calm, relaxed, and peaceful state. Correct physical recovery means to be able to recover from exercises and allow your body to resume its normal function. The key to reaching the mind's calmness and physical body's normal function is through deep and relaxed breathing. Often with the coordination of light massage, you can reach the goals comfortably and naturally.

Tui Na / Acupressure Massage Theory

1. Tui na means "pushing" (tui, 推) and "grabbing" (na, 拿). That means tui na massage uses grabbing, pushing, and rubbing techniques to excite cells and improve qi circulation. Dian xue means "pointing" (dian, 點) and "cavities" (xue, 穴). That means dian xue massage is pointing the pressure in special cavity areas so the qi circulation can be manipulated and improved. Dian xue is commonly called acupressure in Western society. In practice, while tui na massage specializes in leading and spreading the stagnant qi, dian xue specializes in exciting the cells and leading the qi from the deep to the surface around cavity areas.

2. When you massage, remember to keep your fingernails short. If they are too long, not only will you feel uncomfortable when you massage yourself, but you may also scratch and injure yourself.

3. When you massage yourself, especially with acupressure, you should not use too much pressure at the beginning. Pressing the cavity area firmly with adequate pressure is the key of a good stimulation. If the pressure causes too much pain, then the area massaged will be tense, and qi and blood circulation will also be more stagnant.

4. You should know that different cavities and different areas of the body have different sensitivity. You may place a lot of pressure in some cavities and areas and feel stimulated and comfortable, while the same pressure on other cavities and areas will not feel comfortable. For example, the inner thigh area is more sensitive than the external thigh area. Naturally, the level of sensitivity also depends on each individual. Some people are more tolerant of pain than others. Therefore, experience the pressure yourself and see how much pressure you should apply for each cavity. Remember, comfortable and enjoyable pain is good stimulation. Significant pain will only cause qi and blood stagnation.

5. The best routine for massage is to begin from the head and neck, so the mind can be relaxed first. Then follow with the front side of your torso and finally your limbs. In this case, you will use your mind to lead the qi from the center out and also from the top to the bottom.

6. You should know that acupressure is not the same as acupuncture. Acupuncture uses needles to penetrate the body through cavities and reach to the qi channels. It is deep and must be precise. However, in acupressure, because the pressure you apply covers a wider area than acupuncture, you don't have to pinpoint the exact spot of the cavities.

7. Again, feeling is the key to success in acupressure. Through feeling and correct pressure, you will be able to reach the goals of relaxation and stimulation, thus enhancing qi circulation effectively.

8. When these acupressure techniques are applied in the morning right after waking up, the qi circulation in the twelve primary qi channels can be enhanced. However, if you apply these acupressure techniques for the lower limbs right before going to sleep, it will help you fall asleep more easily. This is simply because when you massage your lower limbs, especially your feet, the qi from the upper body will be led downward. This will relax the head and mind. Massaging the feet can also reduce high blood pressure. However, if you massage your head and torso right before sleep, you may experience difficulty in falling sleep because the qi and blood circulation are enhanced in your upper body, especially your head. This may keep you awake.

9. Again, the number of repetitions or the time length of stimulation is only a suggestion. You must experience yourself and adjust accordingly.

10. From some qigong masters' experience, it is suggested that if you have time, you massage these paths and cavities twice per day. This will help you bring your qi circulation to a regulated and healthy level.

3-3. The Network of Qi Vessels and Channels

As explained earlier, we have two bodies: the physical body and the qi body (or bio-electric body). The physical body can be seen, but the qi body can only be felt. The qi body is the vital source of the physical body (i.e., all living cells) and the foundation of our lives. The qi body is not only related to our cells but also to our thinking and shen, because it is the energy source that maintains the brain's functioning. Therefore, any qi imbalance or stagnation will be the root and cause of any physical sickness or mental disorder.

Western medical science has long studied the physical body but for the most part has ignored the qi body. This began to change in the last two decades. Scientific understanding of the qi body, and how it affects our health and longevity, is still in its infancy. Under these circumstances, we may still accept the ancient Chinese understanding of our body's qi network.

Twelve Primary Qi Channels and the Eight Vessels
From the understanding of Chinese medicine, the qi circulatory system in a human body includes eight vessels (ba mai, 八脈), twelve primary qi channels (shi er jing, 十二經), and thousands of secondary channels branching out from the primary channels (luo, 絡). On two of the vessels (conception and governing vessels) (ren and du mai, 督‧任脈) and the twelve primary qi channels, there are more than seven hundred acupuncture cavities, through which the qi level in the channels can be adjusted and regulated. From this qi adjustment, the qi circulation in the body, especially in the internal organs, can be

regulated into a harmonious state, and the body's sickness can be cured and health maintained. Here, we will briefly review these three circulatory networks. If you are interested in learning more about this qi network, you may refer to Chinese acupuncture books or to the book *The Root of Chinese Qigong*, published by YMAA Publication Center.

1. Eight Vessels (Ba Mai) 八脈

A. The eight vessels include four yang vessels and four yin vessels. They balance each other.

B. The four yang vessels are as follows:

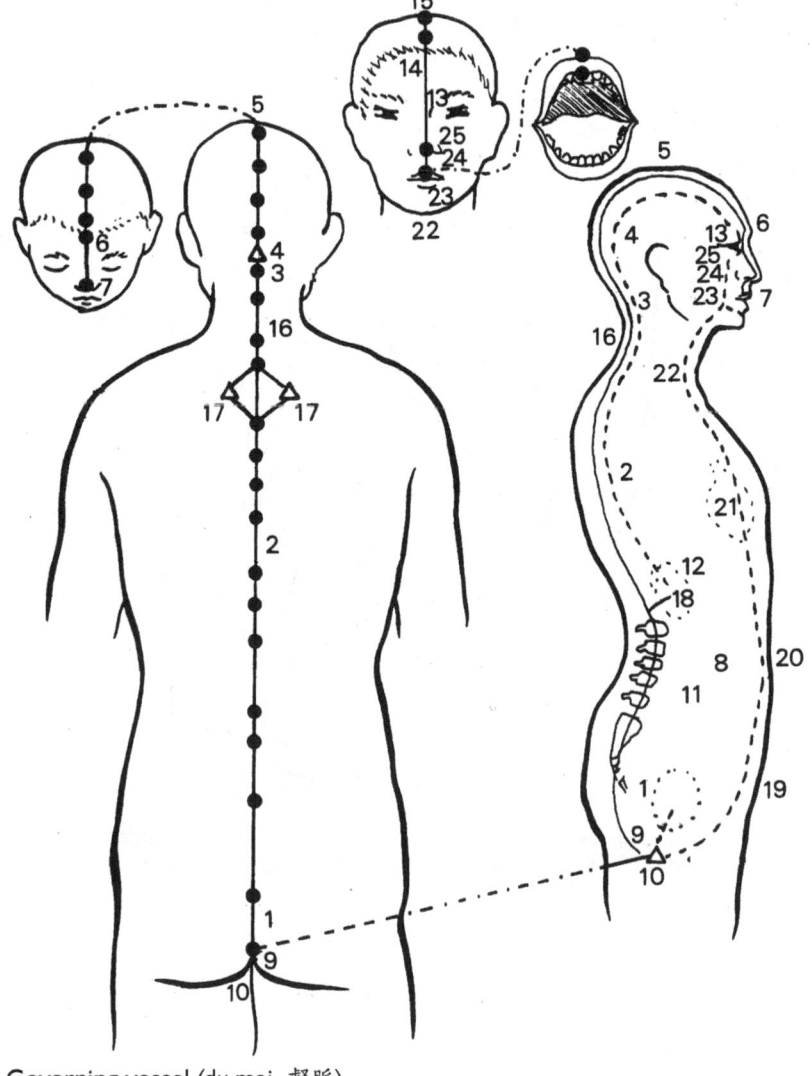

Governing vessel (du mai, 督脈).

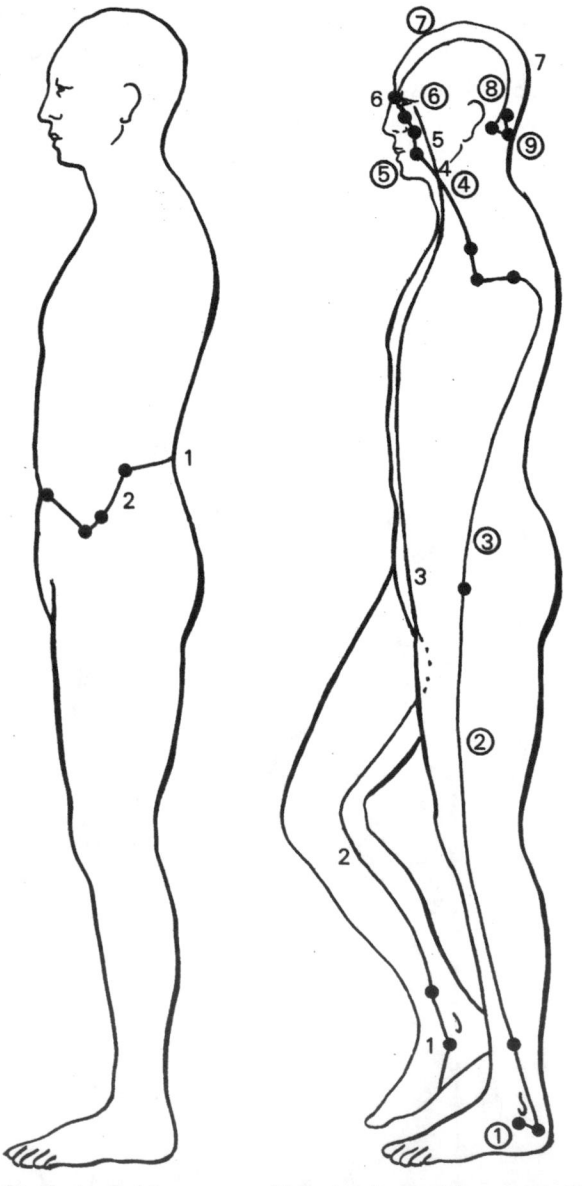

Girdle (or belt)
vessel (dai mai, 帶脈).

Yang heel vessel (external side
of leg) (yangqiao mai, 陽蹻脈).

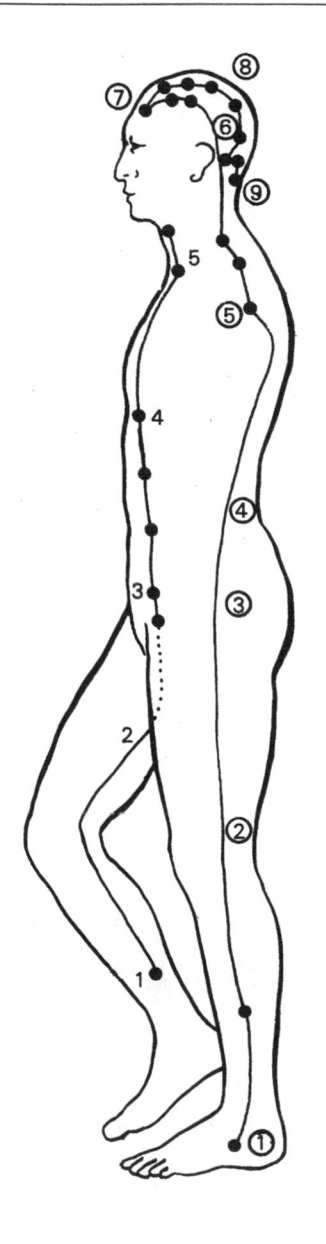

Yang linking vessel (external side of
leg) (yangwei mai, 陽維脈).

The four yin vessels are as follows:

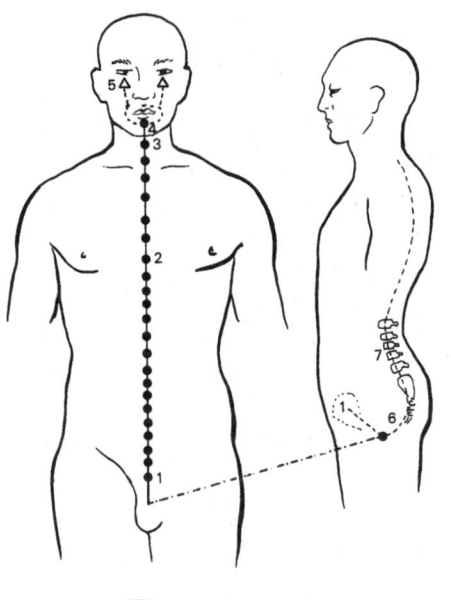

Conception vessel (ren mai, 任脈).

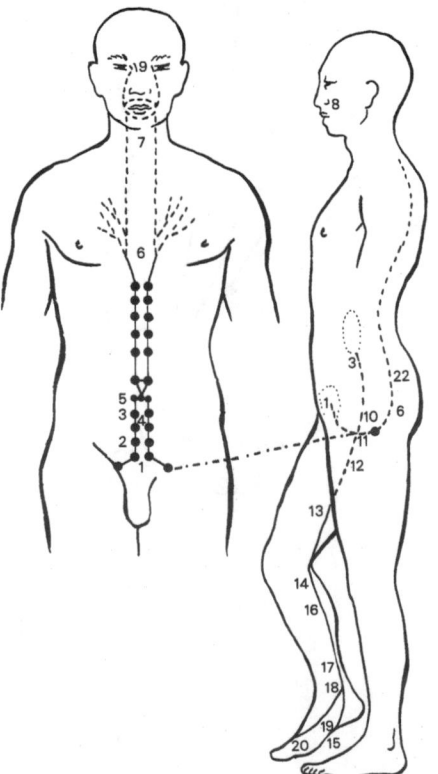

Thrusting vessel (chong mai, 衝脈).

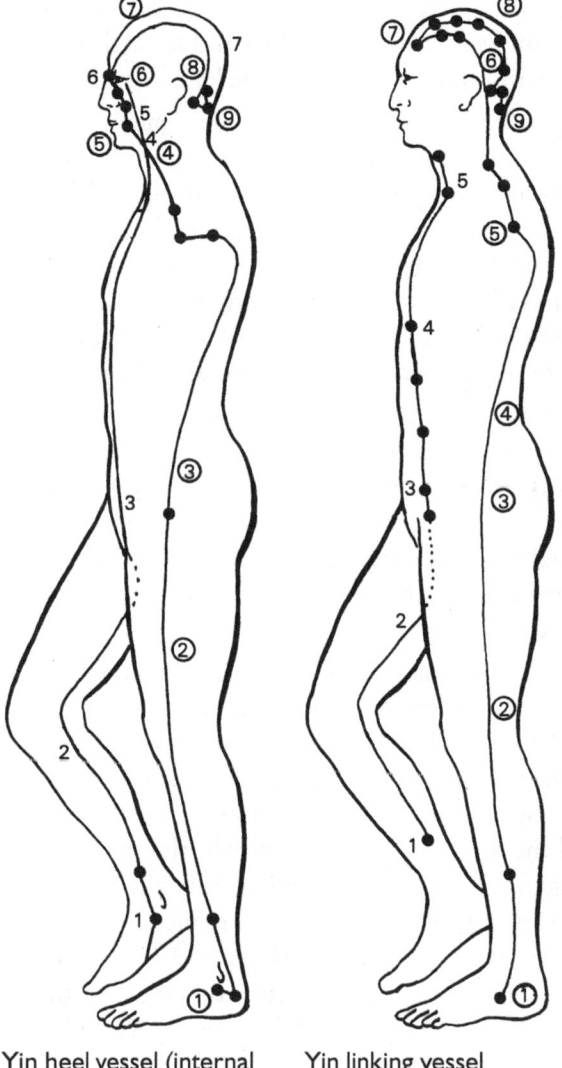

Yin heel vessel (internal side of leg) (yinqiao mai, 陰蹻脈).

Yin linking vessel (internal side of leg) (yinwei mai, 陰維脈).

C. According to Chinese medicine, vessels function as reservoirs, connected to the twelve primary qi channels and regulating the qi level circulating in these channels. When the qi level in some specific channel is too high, one or more of the reservoirs will absorb the excess qi; if the qi is too low, the shortfall will be supplied from these vessels. This enables a harmonious level to be maintained.

D. The two yang vessels (governing and girdle vessels) and the two yin vessels (conception and thrusting vessels) are individual and located in the torso. The other four vessels exist in pairs and are located in the legs. There are no vessels in the arms.

E. Among the eight vessels, according to Chinese medicine, the governing and conception vessels are the most important because they are the main vessels that regulate the twelve primary qi channels. The governing vessel regulates the qi in the six primary yang qi channels, while the conception vessel regulates the qi in the six primary yin qi channels. There are acupuncture cavities on these two vessels but none on the other six vessels. However, there are many cavities on these six vessels that belong to the twelve primary qi channels. These cavities are considered to be gates that allow the qi to pass between the vessels and channels.

F. According to Chinese qigong practice for health and longevity, the methods of learning how to expand the qi in the vessels are very important. The reason for this is that these eight vessels are the reservoirs for the qi. When the qi in these reservoirs is abundant, the qi regulating potential of the primary qi channels will be high and efficient. Among these eight vessels, the governing and conception vessels are the most important because they regulate the twelve primary qi channels. The qi circulates in these two vessels and distributes to the twelve primary qi channels throughout the day.

G. In religious qigong meditation practice for enlightenment, the thrusting vessel (i.e., spinal cord) is very important. The thrusting vessel connects the brain and the perineum, and the qi is abundant in this vessel at midnight. Traditionally, during the midnight hours, we are sleeping, and the physical body is extremely relaxed. In this situation, the physical body does not need a great amount of qi to support its activities, and the qi circulates abundantly in the spinal cord to nourish the brain and sexual organs. Hormone production from the pineal, pituitary, and adrenal glands and the testicles or ovaries is therefore increased at night. When the brain is nourished and its function is raised to a high level, the shen can be raised and enlightenment can be achieved. If you are interested in more on this subject, please refer to the book *Qigong, The Secret of Youth*, published by YMAA Publication Center.

H. The governing vessel, which is located at the center of the back, is the main vessel supplying qi to the nervous system branching out from the spinal cord. The nervous system is constructed of physical cells that need to be nourished with qi (bioelectricity) to function and stay alive. This tells us that qi is ultimately the root of nerve function. To maintain abundant qi circulation in this vessel, your physical condition is extremely important. If there is any physical injury or damage along the course of this vessel, the qi supply to the nervous system will be stagnant and irregular. Moreover, in order to have healthy and abundant qi circulation in this vessel, you must learn how to increase qi storage in the real lower dan tian (zhen xia dan tian, 真下丹田), which is the main qi reservoir or bioelectric battery in our body.

I.   The yang girdle vessel is the only vessel in which the qi circulates horizontally. To qigong practitioners, this vessel is very important. Because the qi status in this vessel is yang, the qi is expanding outward. It is from this vessel that we feel our balance. It is just like an airplane or a tight-rope walker: the longer the wings or the balancing pole, the easier it will be to find and maintain balance. A qigong practitioner or a Chinese martial artist will train this vessel and make the qi expand outward farther, therefore increasing the balance and stability of both the physical and mental bodies. When you have more balance and stability, you can find your center. When you find your physical and mental center, you will be rooted. Once you are rooted, your shen can be raised to a higher level.

2. The Twelve Primary Qi Channels and Their Branches (Shi Er Jing Luo) 十二經絡

A.   The twelve primary qi channels include six yang channels and six yin channels. They balance each other.

B.   The six yang channels are as follows:

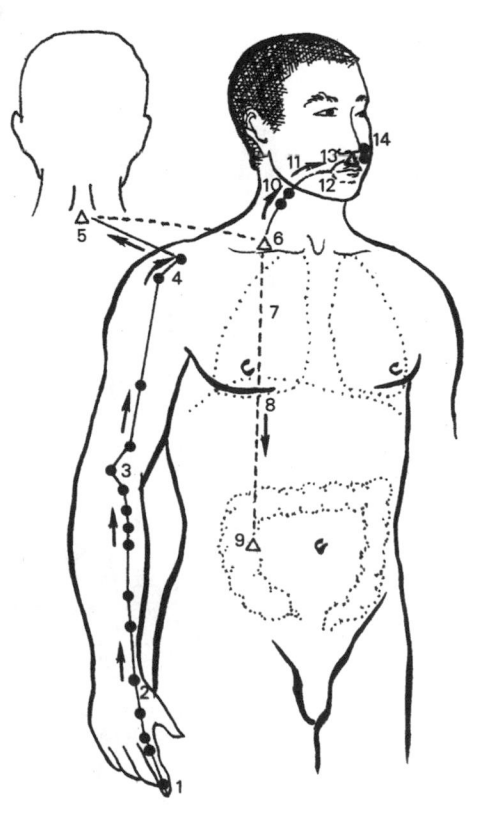

Arm yang brightness large intestine channel (shou yang ming da chang jing, 手陽明大腸經).

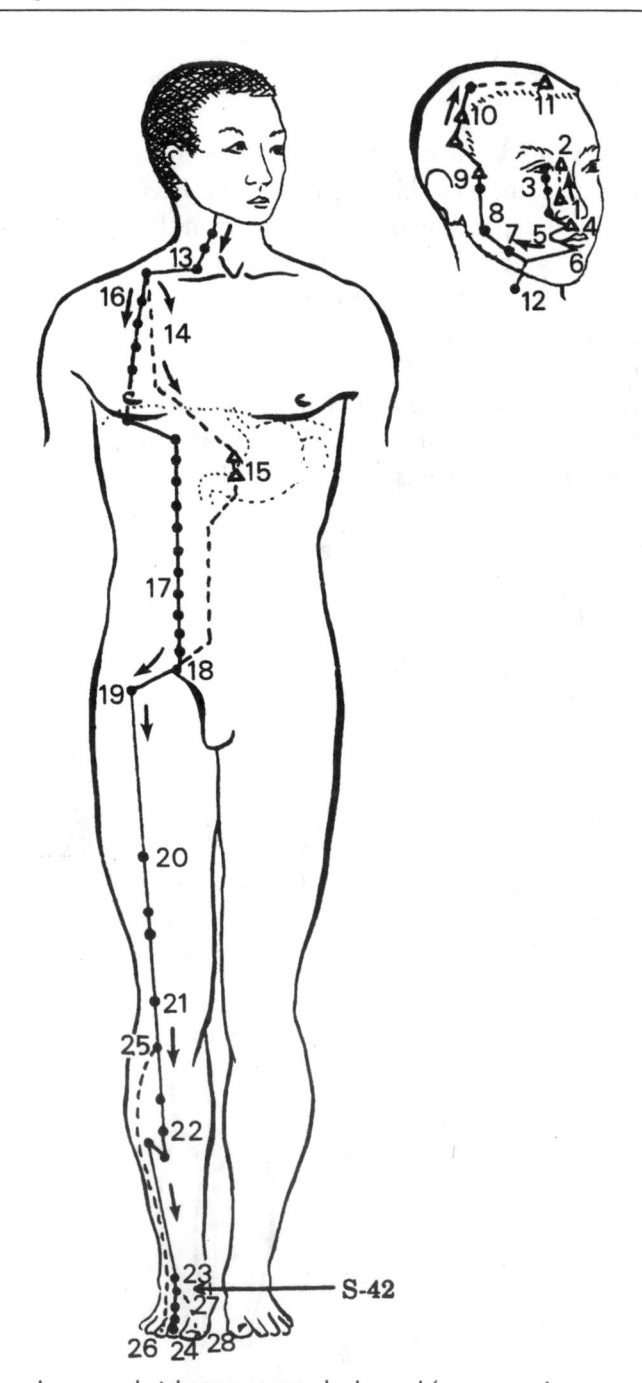

Leg yang brightness stomach channel (zu yang ming wei jing, 足陽明胃經).

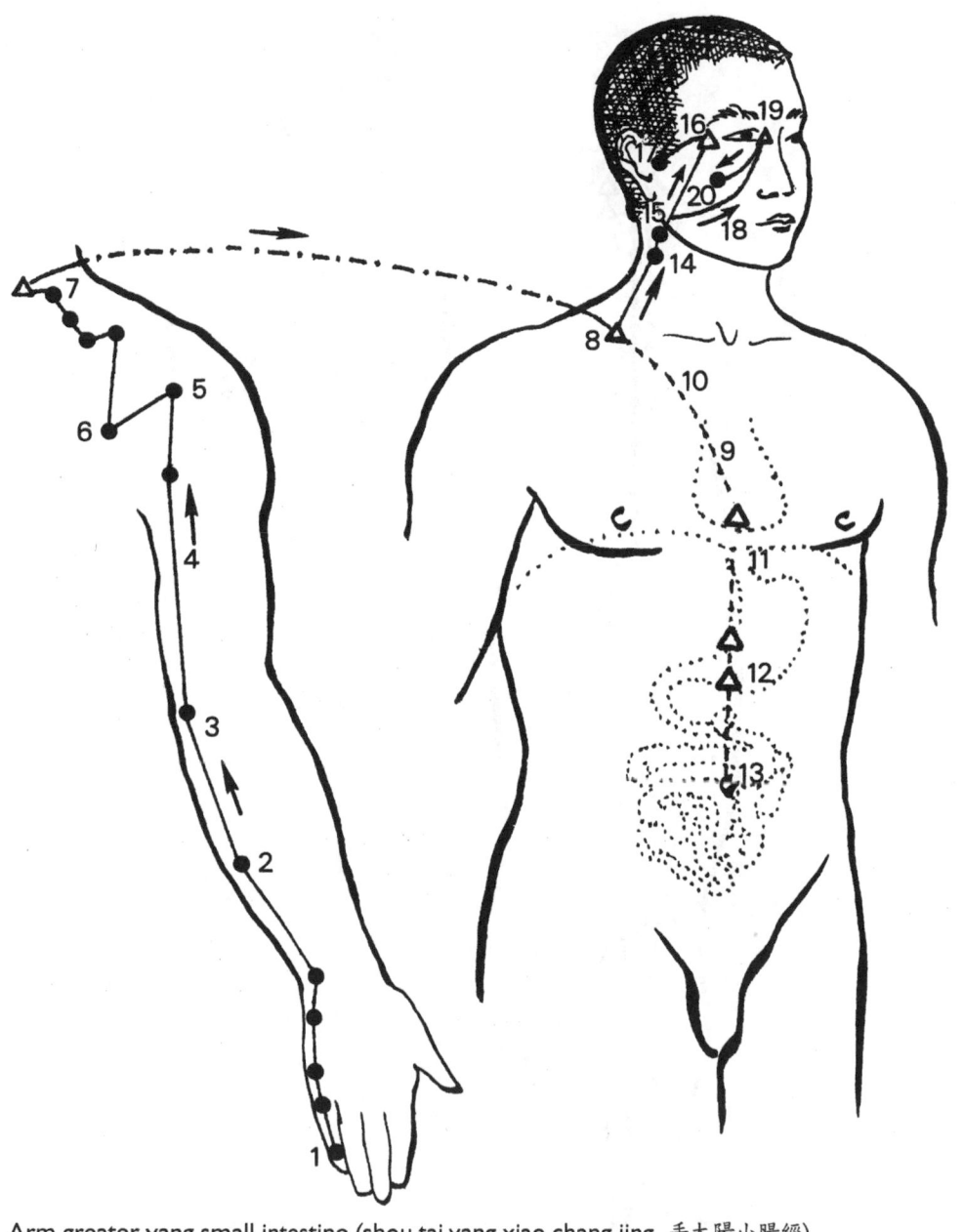

Arm greater yang small intestine (shou tai yang xiao chang jing, 手太陽小腸經).

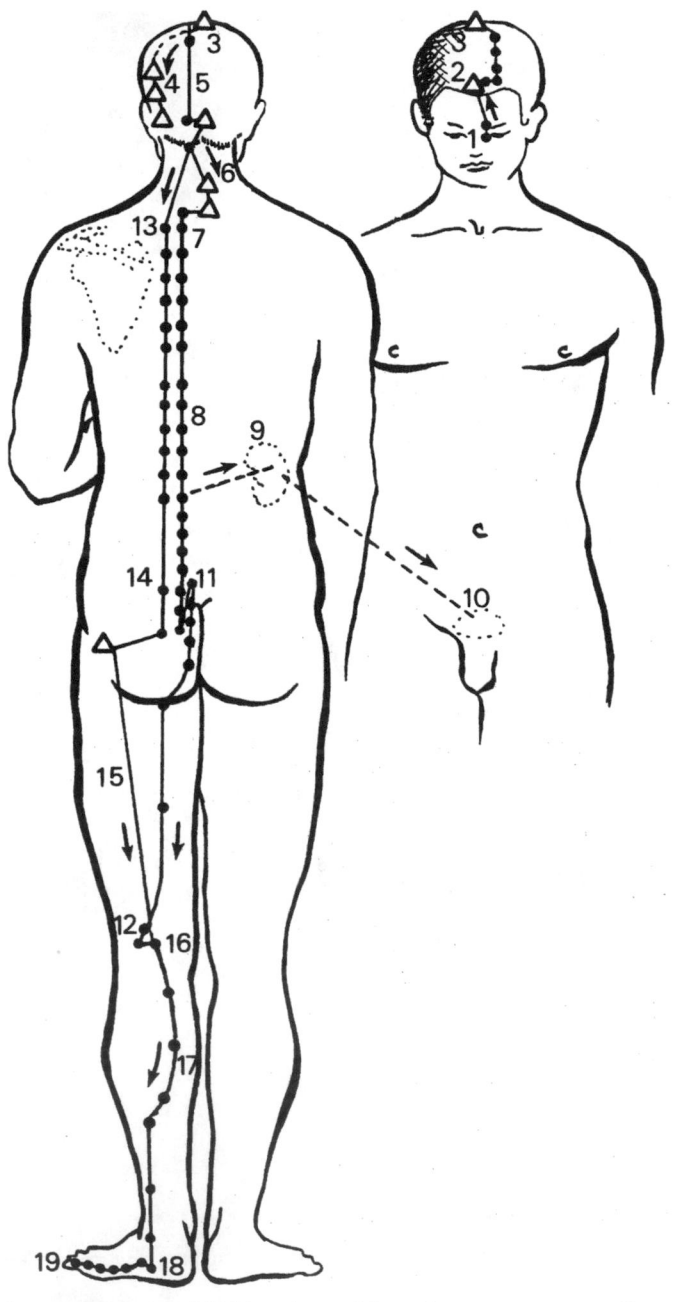

Leg greater yang bladder channel (zu tai yang pang guang jing,
足太陽膀胱經).

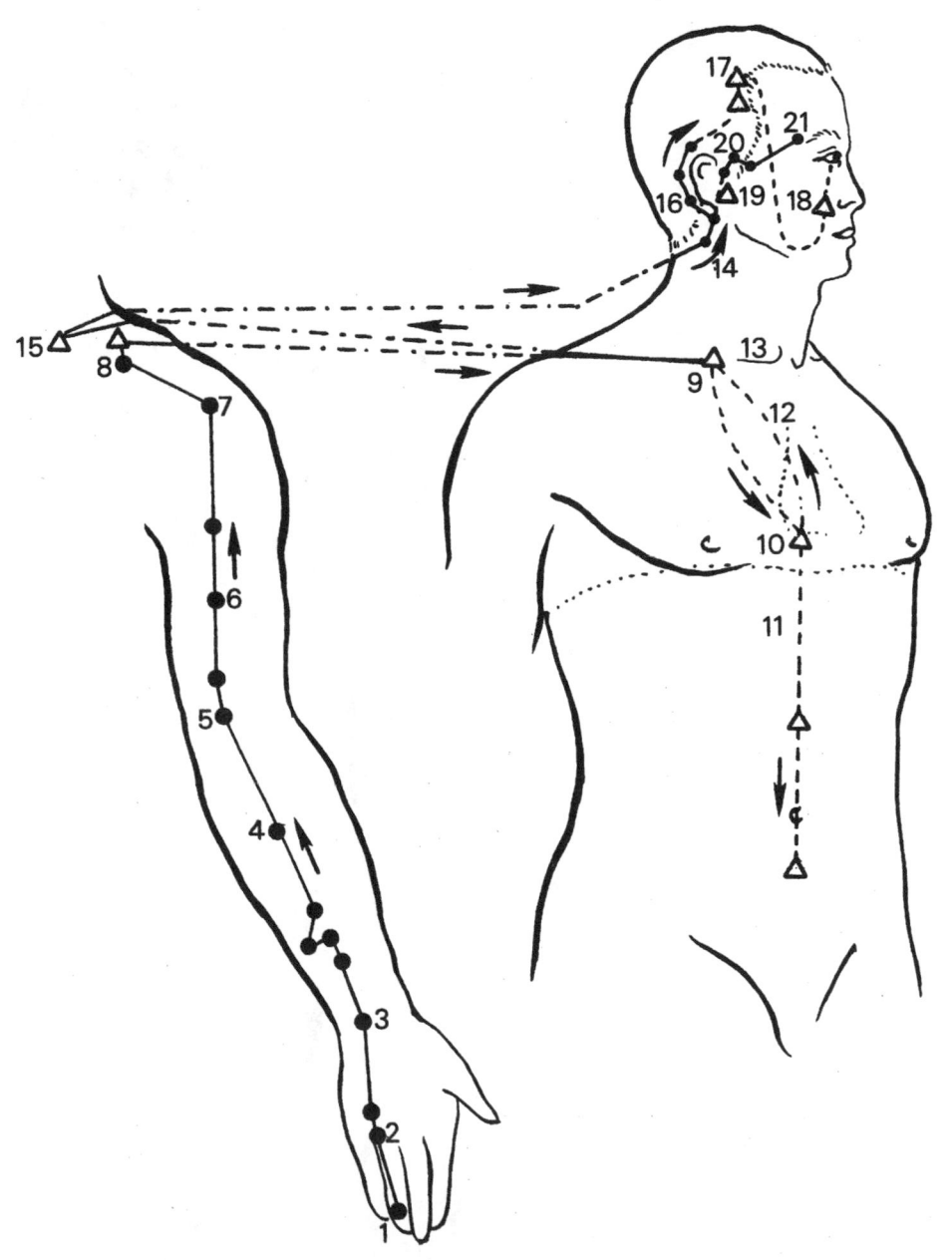

Arm lesser yang triple burner channel (shou shao yang san jiao jing, 手少陽三焦經).

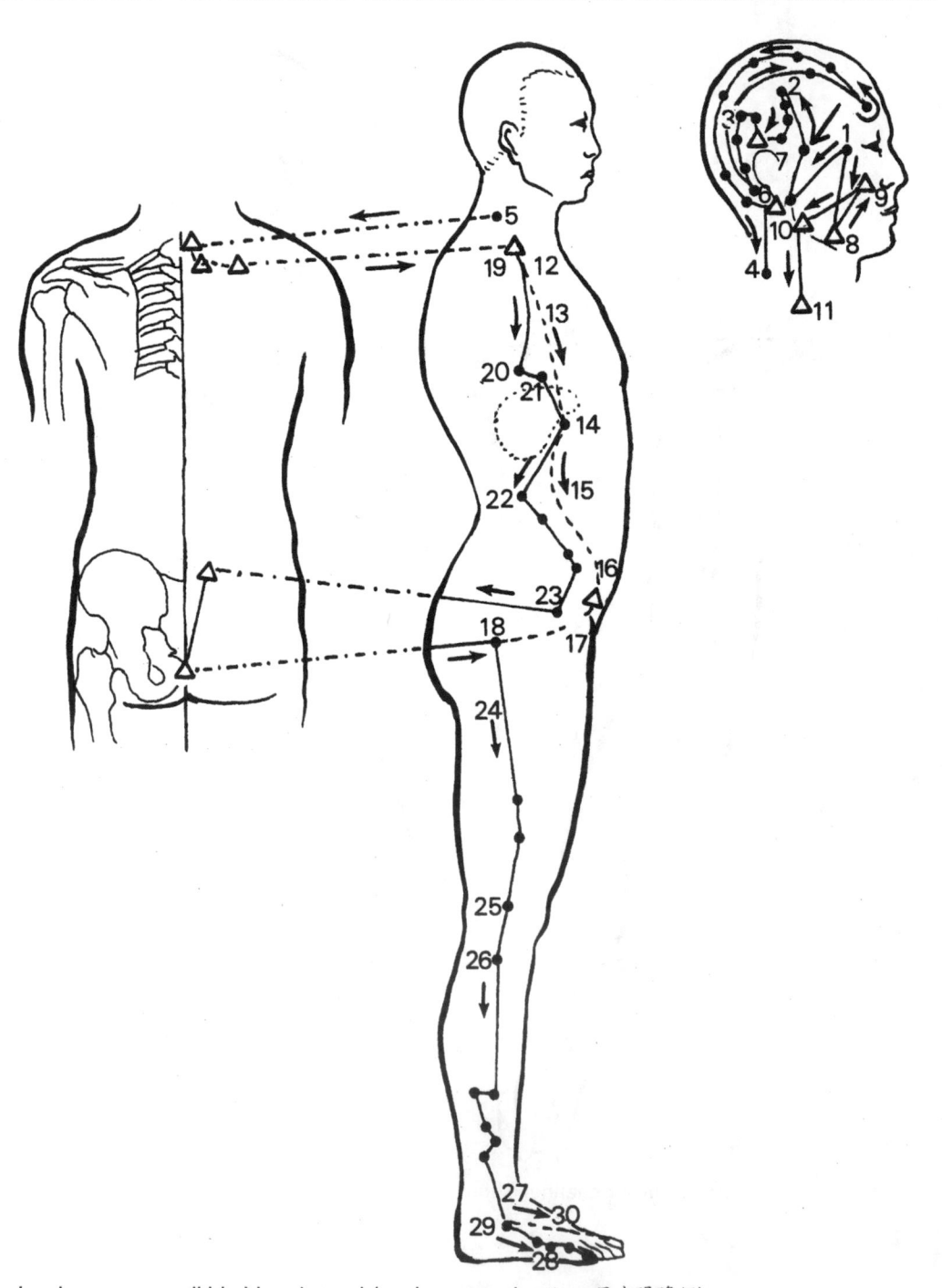

Leg lesser yang gall bladder channel (zu shao yang dan jing, 足少陽膽經).

The six yin channels are as follows:

- ● Points Belonging to Channels
- △ Points of Intersection
- ----- Connecting Lines
- ——— Primary Channels on Which There are Points
- - - - - - Primary Channels and Branches without Points

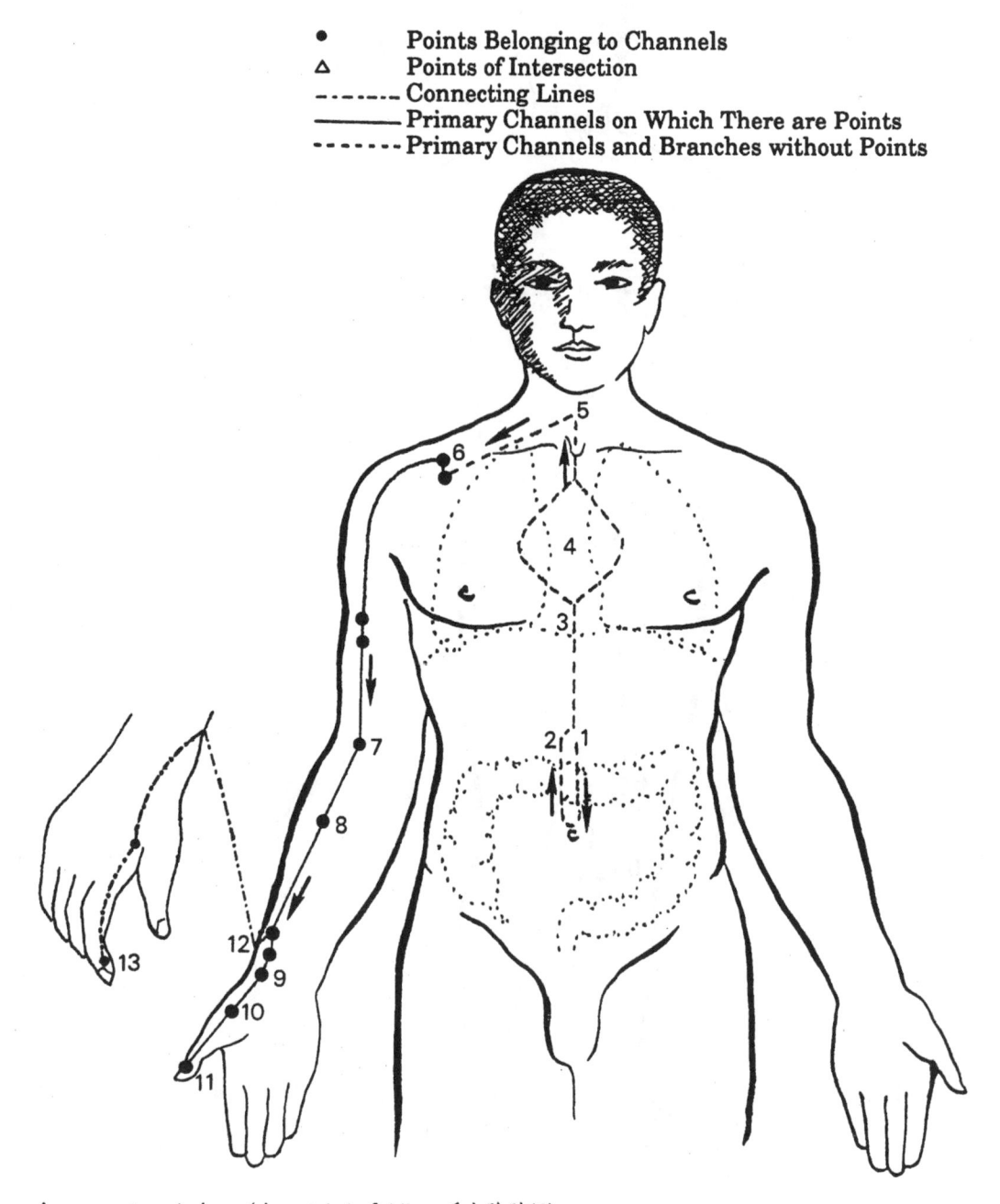

Arm greater yin lung (shou tai yin fei jing, 手太陰肺經).

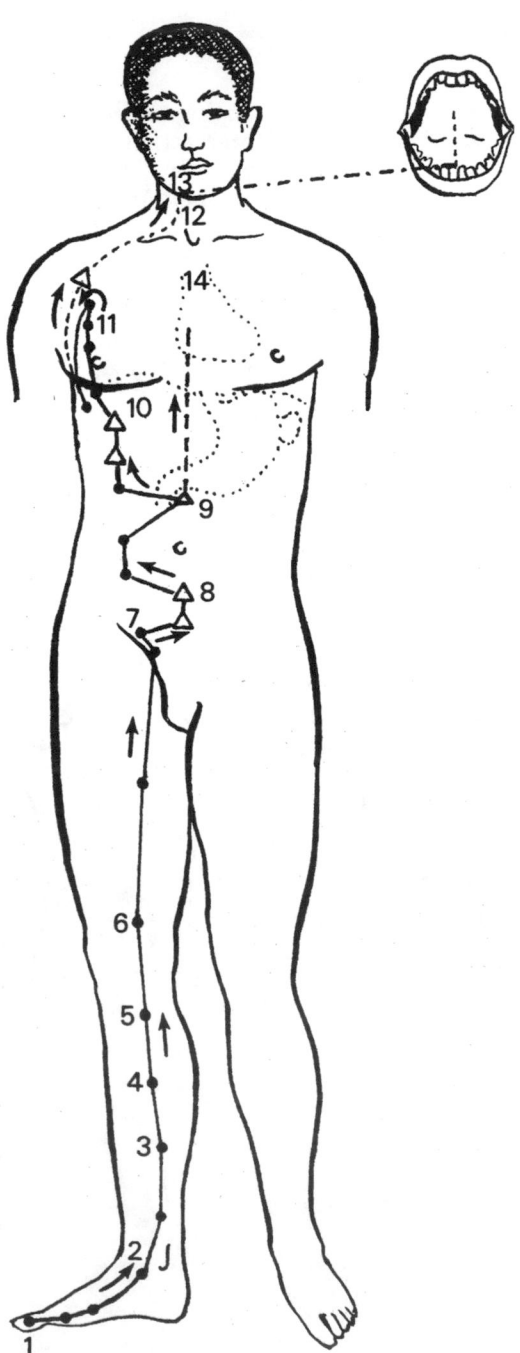

Leg greater yin spleen channel (zu tai yin pi jing,
足太陰脾經).

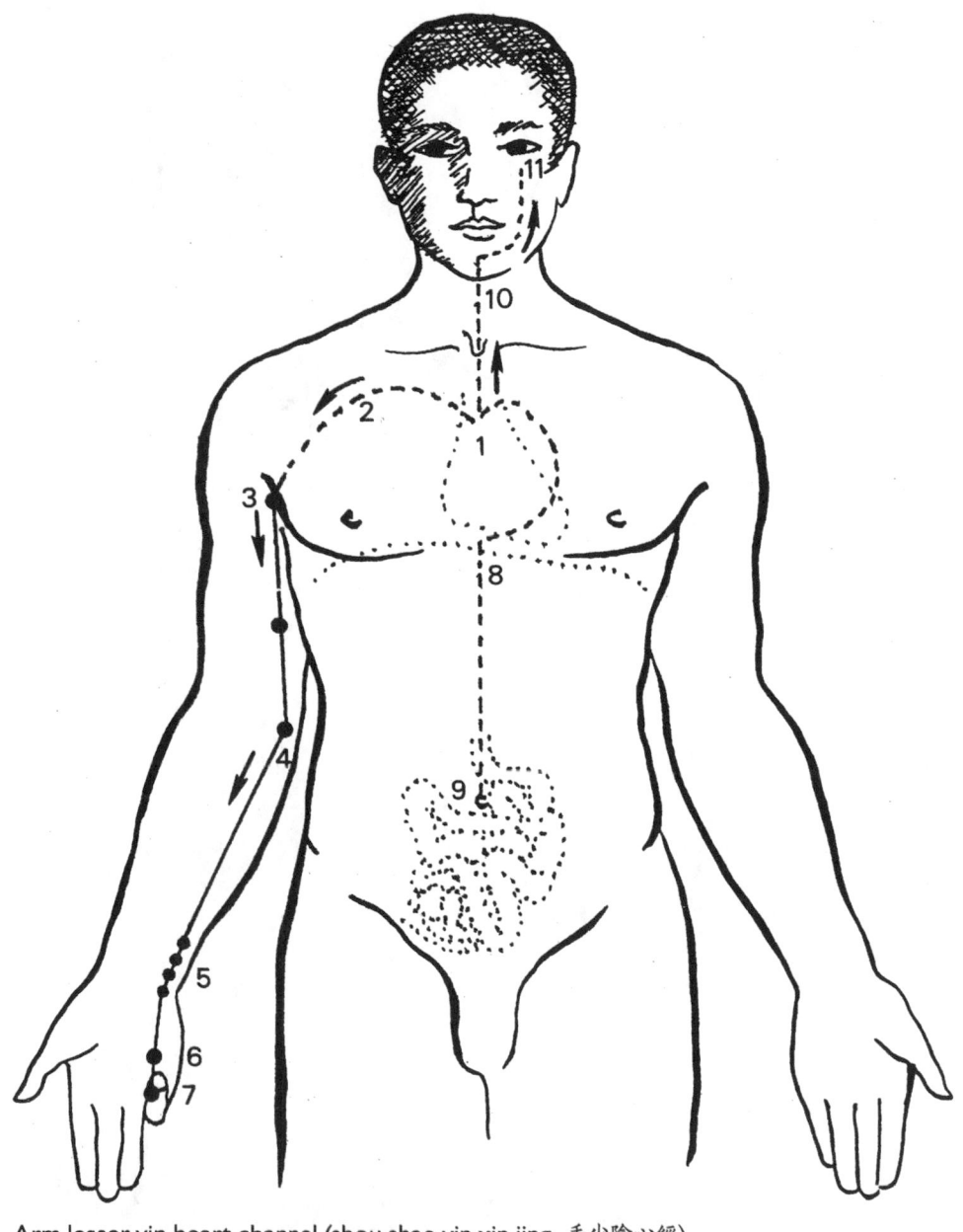

Arm lesser yin heart channel (shou shao yin xin jing, 手少陰心經).

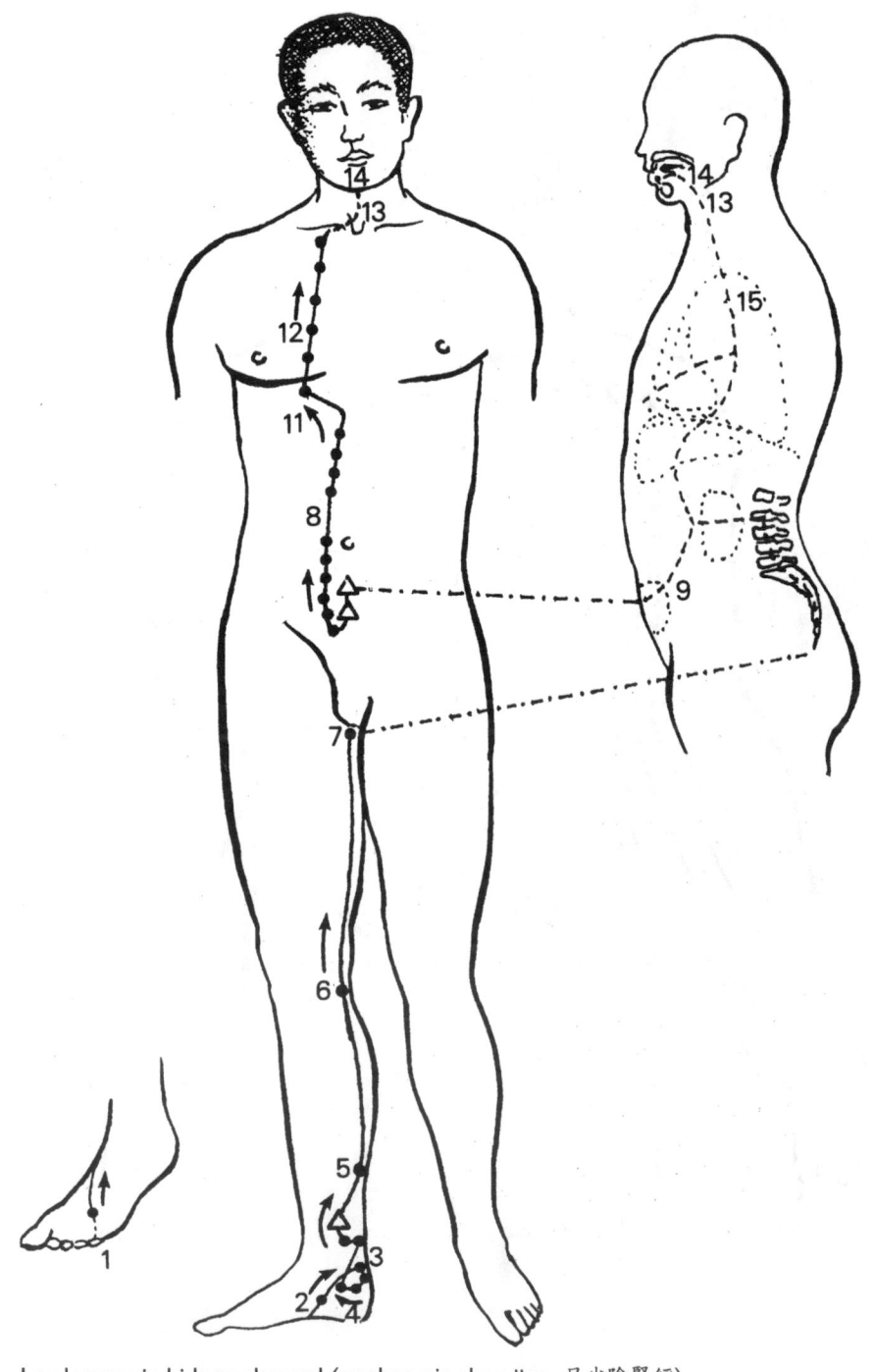

Leg lesser yin kidney channel (zu shao yin shen jing, 足少陰腎經).

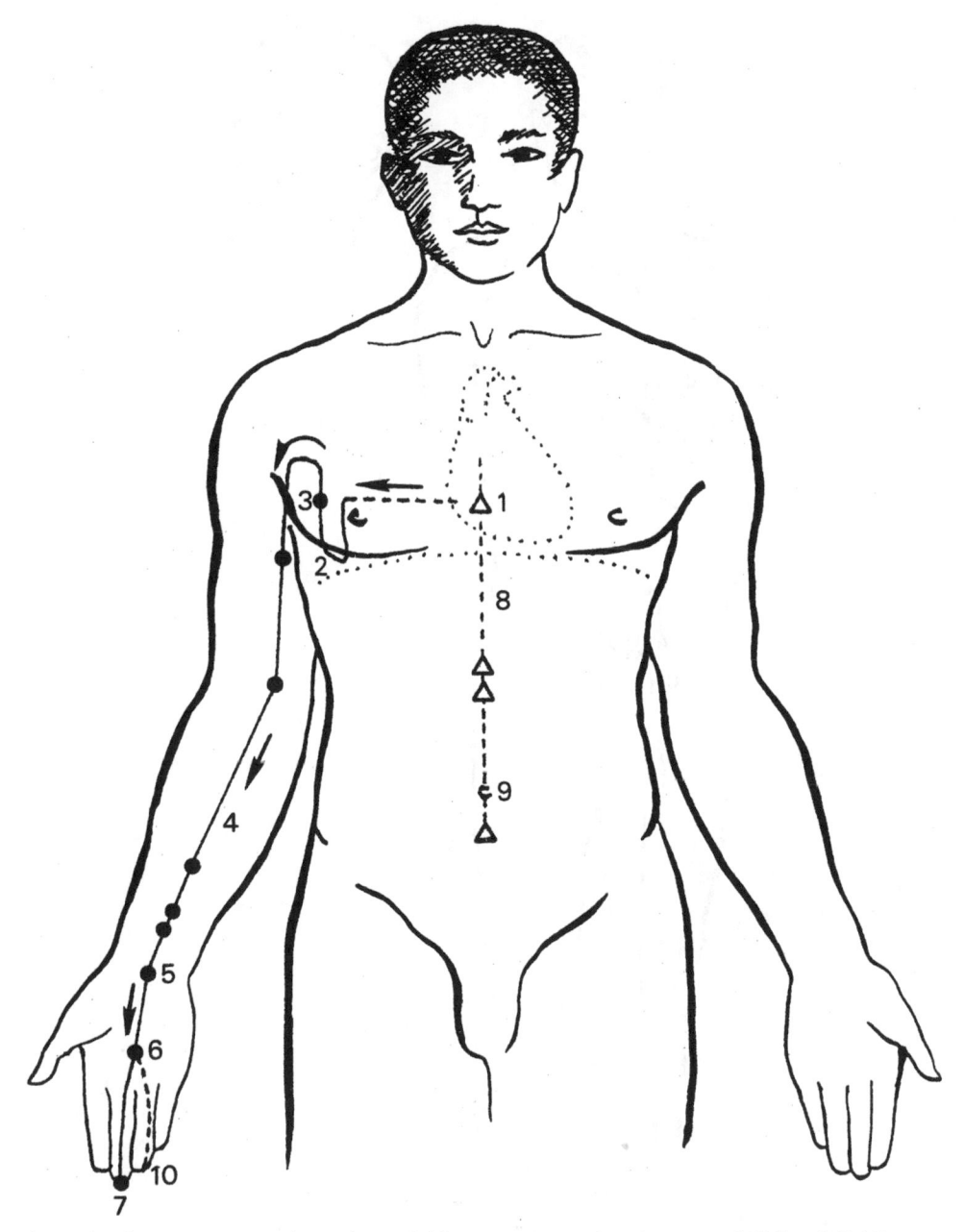

Arm absolute yin pericardium channel (shou jue yin xin bao luo jing, 手厥陰心包絡經).

Leg absolute yin liver channel (zu jue yin gan jing, 足厥陰肝經).

C. From the above, you can see that one end of each channel connects to an extremity, and the other end connects with a different internal organ. In each channel, there are many acupuncture cavities through which the qi condition in each channel can be regulated. This is the basic theory of acupuncture.

D. There are thousands of secondary channels (luo, 絡) branching out from each primary channel; these lead the qi to the surface of the skin and to the bone marrow. It is very similar to the artery and capillary system. Instead of blood, qi is being distributed.

3-4. Buddhist and Daoist Qigong Concepts

Because it was kept so secret, religious qigong did not become as popular as the other categories in China before the Qing dynasty (清朝) (1644–1912 CE). It was not until the twentieth century, when the secrets were gradually released to the public, that religious qigong became popular in China. Religious qigong is mostly Daoist and Buddhist, and its main purpose is to aid in the striving for enlightenment, or what the Buddhists refer to as Buddhahood.

To help you understand both the training theory and methods studied in Buddhist and Daoist societies, I would like to give a brief introduction to Buddhist and Daoist qigong, followed by a comparison of their training.

Buddhist Qigong

Three main schools of Buddhist qigong developed in Asia during the last two thousand years: Indian, Chinese, and Tibetan. Buddhism was created in India between 558 BCE and 478 BCE by an Indian prince named Gautama, and Indian Buddhist qigong has the longest history. Buddhism was imported into China during the Eastern Han dynasty (Dong Han, 東漢) (58 CE), and the Chinese Buddhists learned its methods of spiritual cultivation. Their practice was influenced by traditional Chinese scholars and medical qigong, which had been developing for about two thousand years. What resulted was a unique system of training that was different from its ancestors.

According to the fragments of documents that are available, it is believed that at least in the first few hundred years after Buddhism's importation, only the philosophy doctrines were passed down to the Chinese. The actual methods of cultivation and qigong training were not known. There are several reasons for this:

1. Because of the difficulty of transportation and communication at that time, the transferal of Buddhist documents from India to China was limited. Although a few Indian priests were invited to China to preach, the problems remained.

2. Even if the documents had been transferred, because of the profound theory and philosophy of Buddhism, very few people were qualified and could really translate the documents accurately from Sanskrit to Chinese. This problem was exacerbated by the different cultural backgrounds. Even today, different cultural backgrounds are always the main problem in translating accurately from one language to another.

3. The main reason is probably that most of the actual training methods need to be taught and guided personally by an experienced master. Only a limited amount can be learned from documents. This problem was exacerbated by the tradition of passing information secretly from master to disciples.

You can see that the transfer process was very slow and painful, especially with regard to the actual training methods. For several hundred years, it was believed that as long as you were able to purify your mind and sincerely strive for Buddhahood, sooner or later you would succeed. This situation was not improved until Da Mo (達磨) wrote the *Muscle/Tendon Changing Classic* and the *Marrow/Brain Washing Classic* (*Yi Jin Jing, Xi Sui Jing*; 易筋經、洗髓經). Finally, there was a firm direction for the training to reach the goal of Buddhahood.

Before Da Mo, Chinese Buddhist qigong training was very similar to Chinese scholar qigong. The main difference was that while scholar qigong aimed at maintaining health, Buddhist qigong aimed at becoming a Buddha. Meditation is a necessary process in training a priest to stay emotionally neutral. Buddhism believes that all human spiritual suffering is caused by the seven passions and six desires (qi qing liu yu, 七情六慾). As mentioned earlier, the seven passions are happiness (xi, 喜), anger (nu, 怒), sorrow (ai, 哀), joy (le, 樂), love (ai, 愛), hate (hen, 恨), and desire (yu, 慾). The six desires are the six sensory pleasures derived from the eyes, ears, nose, tongue, body, and mind. Buddhists also cultivate within themselves a neutral state separated from the four emptinesses of earth, water, fire, and wind (si da jie kong, 四大皆空). They believe that this training enables them to keep their spirits independent so they can escape from the cycle of repeated reincarnation.

Tibetan Buddhism has always been kept secret and isolated from the outside world. Because of this, it is very difficult to determine when exactly Tibetan Buddhism was established. Because Tibet is near India, it is reasonable to assume that Tibetan qigong training has had more influence from India than from Chinese qigong. However, over thousands of years of study and research, the Tibetans established their own unique style of qigong meditation. The Tibetan priests are called lamas (la ma, 喇嘛), and many of them also learned martial arts. Because of the different cultural background, not only are the lamas' meditation techniques different from those of the Chinese or Indian Buddhists, but their martial techniques are also different. Tibetan qigong meditation and martial arts were kept secret from the outside world and were therefore called mi zong (秘宗), which means "secret style." Generally speaking, Tibetan qigong and martial arts did not spread into Chinese society until almost the Qing dynasty (清朝) (1644–1912 CE). Since then, however, they have become more popular.

Daoist Qigong

Like the Buddhists, the Daoists believe that if they can build up their shen (神) so that it is independent and strong, they can escape from the cycle of repeated reincarnation. When a Daoist has reached this stage, he has reached the goal of enlightenment. It is said that he has attained eternal life. However, if he cannot build his shen quite strong enough before he dies, his soul or shen will not go to hell, and he can control his own destiny: either remaining a spirit or being reborn as a human. Daoists believe that it is only possible to develop the human spirit while in a body, so that the continual cycle of rebirth is necessary to attain enlightenment.

Daoist monks, in the past, found that in order to enhance their shen, they had to cultivate the qi that was converted from their essence (jing, 精). The normal Daoist qigong training process is (1) to convert the essence (jing) into qi (lian jing hua qi, 練精化氣); (2) to nourish the shen with qi (lian qi hua shen, 練氣化神); (3) to refine the shen and return into nothingness (lian shen fan xu, 練神返虛); and (4) to crush the nothingness (fen sui xu kong, 粉碎虛空).

The first step involved firming and strengthening the jing, then converting this jing into qi through meditation or other methods. This qi is then led to the top of the head to nourish the brain and raise the shen. When a Daoist has reached this stage, it is called the "three flowers meet at the top" (san hua ju ding, 三花聚頂). The three flowers mean essence (jing), qi, and shen. This stage is necessary to gain health and longevity. Finally, the Daoist can start training to reach the goal of enlightenment. However, the biggest obstacle to achieving this goal is the emotions, which affect the thinking and upset the balance of the shen. This is the reason why Daoists hid themselves away in the mountains, away from other people and their distractions. Usually they also abstained from eating meat, feeling that it muddied thinking and increased the emotions, leading the shen away from self-cultivation.

An important part of this training to prolong life is yi jin jing (易筋經) (muscle/tendon changing) and xi sui jing (洗髓經) (marrow/brain washing) qigong. While the yi jin jing qigong is able to build up an abundant qi in the lower dan tian and strengthen the physical body, the basic idea of xi sui jing qigong is to lead the qi to the brain to raise the shen and keep the qi circulating in the marrow so that the marrow stays clean and healthy. Your bone marrow manufactures most of your blood cells. The blood cells bring nourishment to the organs and all the other cells of the body and also take waste products away. When your blood is healthy and functions properly, your whole body is well nourished and healthy and can effectively resist disease. When the marrow is clean and fresh, it manufactures a plentiful quantity of healthy blood cells that will do their job properly.

Your whole body will stay healthy, and the degeneration of your physical body will be significantly slowed.

For longevity, although the theory is simple, the training is very difficult. You must first learn how to build up your qi at the lower dan tian (human biobattery) and fill up your eight qi vessels, and then you must know how to lead this qi into the bone marrow to "wash" the marrow. Except for some Daoist monks, there are very few people who have lived longer than 150 years. The reason for this is that the training process is long and hard. You must have a pure mind and a simple lifestyle so that you can concentrate entirely on the training. Without a peaceful life, your training will not be effective.

Many Daoist qigong styles are based on the theory of cultivating both the shen and the physical body. It is said, "Talking about human temperament [i.e., shen] and life [i.e., physical life], [one] must cultivate both of them. [One must] place the lead [Pb, i.e., yin] and mercury [Hg, i.e., yang] together [i.e., they interact harmoniously]. This message [secret] is hard to comprehend. Cultivating human temperament is to refine self-being, while cultivating life is to return the essence [i.e., convert the essence into qi]. The xin [i.e., mind] is the house of the shen while the body is the residence of the qi. Life is the qi. Those who cultivate human temperament must blend the body and the xin as a family. Jing [essence], qi, and shen must be combined into one unit. Then the cultivation of life can be approached." This paragraph emphasizes that in order to reach enlightenment, you must cultivate both human temperament and physical life. The key to reaching it is to harmonize the yin and yang. Yin is the spiritual body related to human temperament while yang is the physical life related to physical condition. Only when these yin and yang are harmonious and the three treasures (essence, qi, and shen) have reached the top (brain), are you able to achieve the goal of enlightenment.

In Daoism, there are generally three ways of training: golden elixir large way (jin dan da Dao, 金丹大道), dual cultivation (shuang xiu, 雙修), and herb picking outside of the Dao (Dao wai cai yao, 道外採藥). Generally, there are two meanings of dual cultivation: one is to cultivate the qi with a partner, while the other implies both the cultivation of the human temperament and physical body.

Golden elixir large way teaches the ways of qigong training within yourself. This approach believes that you can find the elixir of longevity or even enlightenment within your own body.

In the second approach, dual cultivation, a partner is used to balance one's qi more quickly. Most people's qi is not entirely balanced. Some people are a bit too positive, others too negative, and individual channels are also positive or negative. If you know how to exchange qi with your partner, you can help each other and speed up your training. Your partner can be either the same sex or the opposite.

The third way, herb picking outside of the Dao, uses herbs to speed up and control the cultivation. Herbs can be plants such as ginseng or animal products such as musk from the musk deer. To many Daoists, herbs also mean the qi that can be obtained from sexual practices.

According to the training methods used, Daoist qigong can again be divided into two major schools: peaceful cultivation division (qing xiu paiqing, 清修派) and plant and graft division (zai jie pai, 栽接派). This division was especially clear after the Song and Yuan dynasties (960–1367 CE, 宋、元). The meditation, training theory, and methods of the peaceful cultivation division are close to those of the Buddhists. They believe that the only way to reach enlightenment is golden elixir large way, according to which you build up the elixir within your body. Using a partner for the cultivation is immoral and will cause emotional problems that may significantly affect the cultivation.

However, the plant and graft division claims that their approach of using dual cultivation and herb picking outside of the Dao in addition to golden elixir large way makes the cultivation faster and more practical. For this reason, Daoist qigong training is also commonly called dan ding Dao gong (丹鼎道功), which means the "Dao training in the elixir crucible." The Daoists originally believed that they would be able to find and purify the elixir from herbs. Later, they realized that the only real elixir was in the body.

Acknowledgments

Thanks to Nathan Rosen and Javier Chadud for their photography. Thanks to Rii Kanzaki, Nicholas Yang, Frank Verhülsdonk, Javier Rodriguez, Kyle Olsen, Jonathan Chang, and Enrico Tomei for general help. Thanks to long-term students and friends Bill Buckley, Lisa B. O'Shea for testimonials, and David Silver for a foreword.

Special thank you to my daughter Kathy Yang for her foreword and fact-checking. Her expertise in acupuncture contributed greatly to the accuracy of the information.

Special thanks to everyone at YMAA Publication Center, including T. G. LaFredo for editorial assistance and David Silver for editing the book and companion DVD.

Glossary and Chinese Terms

ai (愛). Kindness, love.

ai (哀). Sorrow.

Ba Duan Jin (八段錦). Eight Pieces of Brocade, wai dan qigong practice created by Marshal Yue, Fei (岳飛) during the Southern Song dynasty (南宋) (1127–1279 CE).

ba kua (八卦). See **bagua**.

ba mai (八脈). The eight vessels of the human body.

bagua (八卦). Eight divinations, also called the eight trigrams. Shown in the *Yi Jing* as groups of single and broken lines. Also called ba kua.

Baguazhang (Ba Kua Chang) (八卦掌). Eight Trigrams Palm. One of the internal qigong martial styles believed to have been created by Dong, Hai-chuan between 1866 and 1880 CE.

Bai He (白鶴). White Crane, one of the Chinese southern martial styles.

baihui (百會, GV-20). Cavity at the top of the head.

baliao (八髎, B-31-34) (仙骨). Cavity of the sacrum.

binao (臂臑, LI-14). Cavity of the biceps.

bu (補). Nourishing process.

Chan (Ren) (禪 or 忍). A Chinese school of Mahayana Buddhism. Asserts that enlightenment can be attained through meditation, self-contemplation, and intuition, rather than through study of scripture. Chan (Ren) is commonly known as Zen in Japan.

chang (長). Long.

Chang Chuan (長拳). See **Changquan**.

changqiang (長強, GV-1) (尾閭). Cavity of the tailbone.

Changquan (長拳). Includes all northern Chinese long-range martial styles.

Chen, Wilson (陳威伸). Dr. Yang, Jwing-Ming's friend.

cheng fo (成佛). Buddhahood.

Cheng, Gin-Gsao (曾金灶). Dr. Yang, Jwing-Ming's White Crane master.

chengshan (承山, BL-57). Cavity on the back of the leg, below the calf muscle.

chi (氣). See **qi**.

chi kung (氣功). See **qigong**.

chin na (擒拿). A component of Chinese martial arts that emphasizes grabbing techniques, to control your opponent's joints, in conjunction with attacking certain acupuncture cavities.

chize (尺澤, LU-5). Cavity of the elbow joint.

chong mai (衝脈). Thrusting vessel. One of the eight extraordinary qi vessels.

Chun Qiu Zhan Guo (春秋戰國). Spring and Autumn Warring Periods, 722–222 BCE.

Confucius (孔子). Chinese philosopher who lived from 551 to 479 BCE. The scholars who practice his philosophy are commonly called Confucians or Confucianists (Ru Jia, 儒家).

Da Mo (達摩). The Indian Buddhist monk, also known as Bodhidharma, who is credited with creating the *Yi Jin Jing* and *Xi Sui Jing* while at the Shaolin monastery. Before he was a monk, his last name was Sardili, prince of a small tribe in southern India.

da zhou tian (大周天). Grand circulation. After a nei dan qigong (內丹氣功) practitioner completes small circulation (xiao zhou tian, 小周天), he will circulate his qi through the entire body or exchange the qi with nature. See **xiao zhou tian; nei dan**.

dan (丹). Elixir.

dan ding Dao gong (丹鼎道功). Literally, Dao training in the elixir crucible. Daoist qigong training.

dan tian (丹田). Locations in the body that can store and generate qi. The upper, middle, and lower dan tian are located respectively between the eyebrows, at the solar plexus, and a few inches below the navel.

Dao (道). The way, by implication, the "natural way."

Dao De Jing (道德經). Morality classic written by Lao Zi (老子). Also written as *Daodejing* and *Tao Te Ching.*

Dao jia (道家). Daoism, as created by Lao Zi during the Zhou dynasty (周) (1122–934 BCE).

Dao wai cai yao (道外採藥). Herb picking outside of the Dao.

di (地). The earth, one of the "three natural powers" (san cai, 三才).

di li shi (地理師). A teacher or master who analyzes geographic locations according to the formulas in the *Book of Changes* (*Yi Jing,* 易經) and the energy distributions in the earth. Di li means "geomancy," and shi means "teacher." See **feng shui shi**.

dian (點). Pointing.

dian mai (點脈). Pointing vessels.

dian qi (電氣). Electric qi.

dian xue (點 穴). Acupressure. Literally, "pointing cavity."

dian xue an mo (點穴按摩). Cavity-press massage.

Dong Han dynasty (東漢). A Chinese dynasty (25–168 CE).

du mai (督脈). The governing vessel, one of the eight extraordinary vessels.

ermen (耳門, TB-21). Cavity in front of the ear. Located above the tinghui (聽會, GB-2).

feng shui (風水). Literally, wind water. The art or science of analyzing the natural energy relationships in a location, especially the interrelationships between wind and water.

feng shui shi (風水師). A wind-water teacher, or master of geomancy, which is the art or science of analyzing the natural energy relationships in a location, especially the interrelationships between wind and water. See **di li shi**.

fengchi (風池, GB-20). Cavity at the base of the skull.

fengfu (風府, GV-16). Cavity at the base of the skull.

fengshi (風市, GB-31). Cavity on the side of the leg.

gongfu (功夫). Energy-time. Anything that takes time and energy to learn or to accomplish is called gongfu. Also known as kung fu.

gongzhong (肱中, EX-UE-21). Cavity on the inside of the upper arm.

gui qi (鬼氣). Ghost qi.

guoshu (國術). Combined and abbreviated form of zhongguo and wushu (中國武術), which means "Chinese martial techniques."

Han dynasty (漢朝). A Chinese dynasty (206 BCE–221 CE).

Han, Ching-Tang (韓慶堂). A well-known Chinese martial artist, especially in Taiwan in the last sixty years. Master Han is also Dr. Yang, Jwing-Ming's Long-Fist grandmaster.

hegu (合谷, LI-4). Cavity in the webbing of the hand. Also known as hukou.

hen (恨). Hate.

Hua Tuo (華佗). Chinese medical doctor credited with creating Five Animal Sports (Wu Qin Xi, 五禽戲).

huantiao (環跳, GB-30). Cavity on the side of the buttock.

huiyin (會陰, CV-1). Acupuncture cavity belonging to the conception vessel (ren mai, 任脈).

hukou (虎口, LI-4). Cavity in the webbing of the hand. Commonly called "tiger mouth." Also known as hegu.

jiache (頰車, ST-6). Cavities on both sides of the jaws, on the cheeks.

jianjing (肩井, GB-21). Cavity between the neck and shoulders.

jiankua (健胯, N-LE-55). Cavity on the side of the hip.

jianneiling (肩內陵, M-UE-48). Cavity at the front of the shoulder.

jianyu (肩髃, LI-15). Cavity located at the shoulder joint.

jiexi (解谿, ST-41). Cavity of the ankle.

jimen (箕門, SP-11). Cavity on the inside of the upper thigh.

Jin, Shao-Feng (金紹峰). Dr. Yang, Jwing-Ming's White Crane grandmaster.

jin dan da Dao (金丹大道). Golden elixir large way.

jin zhong zhao (金鐘罩). Golden bell cover. Also called iron shirt (tie bu shan, 鐵布衫).

jing (精). Essence. The most refined part of anything.

jing (靜). Calm and silent.

jing (經). Called channels but also translated as meridian. Refers to the twelve organ-related "rivers" that circulate qi throughout the body.

jingming (睛明, BL-1). Cavity located where the inner part of the eye meets the nose. Also known as the inner canthus.

jing qi (精氣). Essence qi, which has been converted from original essence.

jiuwei (鳩尾, CV-15). Cavity on the lower sternum.

Jun Qing (君倩). A Daoist and Chinese doctor from the Chinese Jin dynasty (265–420 CE, 晉). Credited as the creator of Five Animal Sports qigong (Wu Qin Xi, 五禽戲).

Kao, Tao (高濤). Dr. Yang, Jwing-Ming's first taijiquan master.

kan (坎). In qigong kan represents water.

kan-li (坎離). In qigong, "water-fire."

kong qi (空氣). Space energy.

kongzui (孔最, LU-6). Cavity of the inner arm.

kufang (庫房, ST-14). Cavity at the front of the shoulder.

kung (功). See **gong**.

kung fu (功夫). See **gongfu**.

kuoshu (國術). National techniques, another name for Chinese martial arts. First used by President Chiang, Kai-Shek (蔣介石) in 1926 at the founding of the Nanking Central Guoshu Institute (南京中央國術館). See **guoshu**.

la ma (喇嘛). A Tibetan priest.

Lao Zi (Li, Er) (老子). The creator of scholarly Daoism, nicknamed Li, Er (李耳).

laogong (勞宮, PC-8). Cavity of the palm.

le (樂). Joy.

li (離). In qigong li represents fire.

Li, Mao-Ching (李茂清). Dr. Yang, Jwing-Ming's Long Fist master.

Li, Shi-Zhen (李時珍). Famous Chinese Daoist medical doctor. Author of *The Study of Strange Meridians and Eight Vessels* (*Qi Jing Ba Mai Kao*, 奇經八脈考).

lian jing hua qi (練精化氣). Convert the essence (jing) into qi.

lian shen fan xu (練神返虛). To refine the shen and return into nothingness.

lian qi (練氣). To train qi. Refers to the belief that it is possible to train your qi to make it stronger and to extend your life.

lian qi hua shen (練氣化神). Nourish the shen (spirit) with qi.

Liang dynasty (梁). A Chinese dynasty (502–557 CE).

lieque (列缺, LU-7). Cavity of the inner arm, just above the wrist.

luo (絡). The small qi channels that branch out from the primary qi channels and are connected to the skin and to the bone marrow.

mai (脈). Vessel or qi channel.

na (拿). Grab.

nei (內). Internal.

nei dan (內丹). A form of qigong in which qi (the elixir) is built up in the body and spread out to the limbs.

nei shi gongfu (內視功夫). Nei shi means to look internally, so nei shi gongfu refers to the art of looking inside yourself to read the state of your health and the condition of your qi.

neiguan (內關, PC-6). Cavity of the inner arm, above the wrist.

nu (怒). Anger.

ping (平). Peace.

quan rou (圈揉). Circular rubbing motion.

qi (氣). Qi is universal energy, including heat, light, and electromagnetic energy. Qi also refers to the energy circulating in human and animal bodies. A current popular model is that the qi circulating in the human body is bioelectric in nature. Also written "chi."

Qi Hua Lun (氣化論). *Qi Variation Thesis.* An ancient treatise that discusses the variations of qi in the universe.

Qi Jing Ba Mai Kao (奇經八脈考). *The Study of Strange Meridians and Eight Vessels.* Book by Li, Shi-Zhen (李時珍), a famous Chinese Daoist medical doctor.

qi qing liu yu (七情六慾). The seven passions and six desires. The seven passions are happiness (xi, 喜), anger (nu, 怒), sorrow (ai, 哀), joy (le, 樂), love (ai, 愛), hate (hen, 恨), and desire (yu, 慾). The six desires are the six sensory pleasures derived from the eyes, ears, nose, tongue, body, and mind.

qi shi (氣勢). Energy state.

qigong (氣功). Gong means gongfu (energy-time). Qigong means study, research, and practices related to qi. Also spelled "chi kung."

qihaishu (氣海俞, BL-24). Cavity of the lower back, alongside the spine.

qihu (氣戶, ST-13). Cavity at the front of the shoulder.

qin na (擒拿). See **chin na**.

Qing dynasty (清朝). The last Chinese dynasty (1644–1912 CE).

qing xiu pai (清修派). The peaceful cultivation division of Daoist qigong training that is similar to that of Buddhism.

quchi (曲池, LI-11). Cavity of the biceps.

quze (曲澤, PC-3). Cavity of the elbow joint.

re qi (熱氣). Heat qi.

ren (仁). Humanity.

ren (人). Man or mankind.

Ren (Chan) (禪 or 忍). A Chinese school of Mahayana Buddhism. Asserts that enlightenment can be attained through meditation, self-contemplation, and intuition, rather than through study of scripture. Chan (Ren) is commonly known as Zen in Japan.

ren mai (任脈). Conception vessel, one of the eight extraordinary vessels.

ren qi (人氣). Human qi.

ren shi (人事). Human events, activities, and relationships.

renzhong (人中, GV-26). The cavity beneath the nose. Also called shuigou (水溝).

Ru Jia (儒家). Confucians or Confucianists.

ruan quan (軟拳). Soft styles.

rugen (乳根, ST-18). Cavity on the front of the chest, behind the nipple.

ruzhong (乳中, ST-17). Cavity on the front of the chest, below the nipple.

san cai (三才). Three powers: heaven, earth, and man.

san gong (散功). An energy problem.

san hua ju ding (三花聚頂). Three flowers meet at the top. A stage of qigong training that is necessary to gain health and longevity. The term "three flowers" refers to essence (jing), qi, and spirit (shen).

sanjiao (三焦). The triple burner. In Chinese medicine, the body is divided into three sections: the upper burner (shang jiao, 上焦) (chest); the middle burner (zhong jiao, 中焦) (stomach area); and the lower burner (xia jiao, 下焦) (lower abdomen).

sanyinjiao (三陰交, SP-6). Cavity on the inside of the leg, above the ankle.

shangwan (上脘, CV-13). Cavity below the sternum.

shanzhong (膻中, CV-17). Cavity on the upper sternum.

Shaolin Temple (少林寺). A monastery located in Henan Province (河南省). Well known for its martial arts training.

shen (神). Spirit. According to Chinese qigong, the shen resides at the upper dan tian (shang dan tian, 上丹田) and is called the third eye.

shen (深). Deep.

shen qi xiang he (神氣相合). Shen and qi mutually combined or harmonized.

shen tong (神通). Enlightenment.

shen xi (神息). Shen breathing.

shen xi xiang yi (神息相依). Shen (spirit) and breathing depend on each other.

shenshu (腎俞, B-23). An acupuncture cavity belonging to the bladder qi channel (膀胱經).

shenting (神庭, GV-24). Cavity in the center of the forehead.

shi er jing (十二經). Twelve major qi channels, or meridians.

shi er jing luo (十二經絡). Twelve primary qi channels and their branches.

shou jue yin xin bao luo jing (手厥陰心包絡經). Arm absolute yin pericardium channel.

shou shao yang san jiao jing (手少陽三焦經). Arm lesser yang triple burner channel.

shou shao yin xin jing (手少陰心經). Arm lesser yin heart channel.

shou tai yang xiao chang jing (手太陽小腸經). Arm greater yang small intestine.

shou tai yin fei jing (手太陰肺經). Arm greater yin lung.

shou yang ming da chang jing (手陽明大腸經). Arm yang brightness large intestine channel.

shousanli (手三里, LI-10). Cavity of the inner arm, near the elbow joint.

shuang xiu (雙修). Dual cultivation.

shuigou (水溝). The cavity beneath the nose. Also called renzhong (人中, GV-26).

si da jie kong (四大皆空). The four emptinesses of earth, water, fire, and wind.

si qi (死氣). Dead qi.

Song dynasty (宋朝). Chinese dynasty (960–1279 CE).

Southern Song dynasty (南宋). After the Song dynasty was conquered by the Jin race from Mongolia, the Song people moved to the south and established another country, called Southern Song, from 1127–1279 CE.

suan ming shi (算命師). Calculate-life teacher. A fortuneteller who is able to calculate a person's future and destiny.

tie bu shan (鐵布衫). Iron shirt. Also called **jin zhong zhao** (金鐘罩), or golden bell cover.

tai chi chuan (taijiquan) (太極拳). A Chinese internal martial style based on the theory of taiji (grand ultimate, 太極).

taichong (太衝, LR-3). Cavity of the top of the foot.

taiji (太極). Grand ultimate. The force that generates two poles, yin and yang.

taixi jing zuo (胎息靜坐). Embryonic breathing meditation.

taiyang (太陽, EX-HN-5). The left temple. Taiyin is on the right temple.

taiyin (太陰, EX-HN-5). The right temple. Taiyang is on the left temple.

taizuquan (太祖拳). A style of Chinese external martial arts.

tian (天). Heaven or sky.

tian qi (天氣). Heaven qi. It is now commonly used to mean the weather, since weather is governed by heaven qi.

tian ren he yi (天人合一). To unify the natural spirit and human spirit.

tian shi (天時). Heavenly timing. The repeating natural cycles generated by the heavens, such as seasons, months, days, and hours.

tian yan (天眼). The heaven eye.

tianzhu (天柱, BL-10). Cavity at the base of the skull.

tiao xin (調心). To regulate the emotional mind.

tinghui (聽會, GB-2). Cavity in front of the ear. Located below the ermen (耳門, TB-21)

tie bu shan (鐵布衫). Gongfu training that toughens the body externally and internally is called "iron shirt."

tu-na (吐納). To "utter and admit," which implies uttering and admitting the air through the nose.

tui (推). Push.

tui na (推拿). "To push and grab." A category of Chinese massage for treating injuries and promoting healing.

wai dan (外丹). External (elixir) qigong exercises in which a practitioner will build up the qi in the limbs and then lead it into the center of the body for nourishment.

weizhong (委中, BL-40). Cavity directly behind the knee joint.

Wu Qin Xi (五禽戲). Five Animal Sports, a medical qigong practice created by Jun Qing (君倩) during the Chinese Jin dynasty (晉) (265–420 CE).

wushu (武術). A common name for the Chinese martial arts. Many other terms are used, including (wuyi, 武藝), for martial arts; (wugong, 武功) for martial gongfu; (guoshu, 國術), for national techniques; and (gongfu, 功夫), which refers to energy-time. Because wushu has been modified into gymnastic martial performance in mainland China over the past forty years, many traditional Chinese martial artists have given up the name "wushu" to avoid confusing modern wushu with traditional wushu. Recently, mainland China has attempted to return modern wushu to its traditional training and practice.

xi (喜). Happiness.

Xi Sui Jing (洗髓經). *Washing Marrow/Brain Classic*, usually translated "*Marrow/Brain Washing Classic.*" Qigong training that specializes in leading qi to the marrow to cleanse it or to the brain to nourish the spirit for enlightenment. It is believed that Xi Sui Jing training is the key to longevity and achieving spiritual enlightenment.

xia dan tian (下丹). Lower dan tian. Located in the lower abdomen, the lower dan tian is believed to be the residence of water qi and original qi.

xiao (孝). Filial piety.

xiao zhou tian (小周天). Called small heavenly cycle, also called small circulation. In qigong, when you can use your mind to lead qi through the conception and governing vessels (任， 督脈), you have completed the cycle.

xiawan (下脘, CV-10). Cavity above the naval.

xie (洩). Energy.

ximen (郤門, PC-4). Cavity of the forearm.

xin (信). Trust.

xin (心). Heart. Also, the "fire mind"—a yang mind or emotional mind.

xiu (修). To regulate.

xiu qi (修氣). Cultivating qi.

Xingyiquan (hsing yi chuan) (形意拳). "Shape-mind fist." An internal style of gongfu in which the mind or thinking determines the shape or movement of the body. Creation of the style is attributed to Marshal Yue, Fei (岳飛).

Xinzhu Xian (新竹縣). Birthplace of Dr. Yang, Jwing-Ming in Taiwan.

xue (血). Blood.

xue (穴). Cavity.

xuehai (血海, SP-10). Cavity of the thigh, near the knee.

yang (陽). In Chinese philosophy, this is the active, positive, masculine polarity. In Chinese medicine, yang means excessive, overactive, overheated. The yang (or outer) organs are the gall bladder, small intestine, large intestine, stomach, bladder, and triple burner.

Yang, Jwing-Ming (楊俊敏). Author of this book.

yanglingquan (陽陵泉, GB-34). Cavity of the back of the leg, below the knee.

yangchi (陽池, TB-4). Cavity of the wrist.

yangqiao mai (陽蹻脈). Yang heel vessel.

yangwei mai (陽維脈). Yang linking vessel.

yi (意). Harmony. Also, the "water mind." The mind of clear thinking and judgment, which is able to make you calm, peaceful, and wise.

yifeng (翳風, TB-17). Cavity behind the base of the ear.

Yi Jin Jing (易筋經). *The Changing Muscle/Tendon Classic*, credited to Da Mo. Written around 550 CE, this work discusses wai dan qigong training for strengthening the physical body.

Yi Jing (易經). *Book of Changes*. A book of divination written during the Zhou dynasty (周) (1122–934 BCE).

yin (陰). In Chinese philosophy, this is the passive, negative, feminine polarity. In Chinese medicine, yin means deficient. The yin (internal) organs are the heart, lungs, liver, kidneys, spleen, and pericardium.

ying gong (硬功). Hard gong. Hard qigong training.

yingchuang (膺窗, ST-16). Cavity on the front of the chest, above the nipple.

yingxiang (迎香, LI-20). The cavity beside the nose.

yinlingquan (陰陵泉, SP-9). Cavity on the back of the leg, above the calf muscle.

yinqiao mai (陰蹻脈). Yin heel vessel.

yintang (印堂, EX-HN-3). The cavity between the eyes. Known as the third eye.

yinwei mai (陰維脈). Yin linking vessel.

yongquan (湧泉, K-1). Cavity of the foot. Called the bubbling well, it is an acupuncture cavity belonging to the kidney primary qi channel.

yu (慾). Desire.

Yuan dynasty (元代). A Chinese dynasty (1206–1367 CE).

yuan qi (元氣). Original qi. Created from the original essence inherited from a person's parents.

Yue, Fei (岳飛). A Chinese military hero from the Southern Song dynasty (南宋) (1127–1279 CE). He is said to have created Ba Duan Jin (八段錦), Xingyiquan (形意拳), and Yue's Ying Zhua (岳家鷹爪).

yujia (瑜珈). Yoga.

zai jie pai (栽接派). Plant and graft division.

zanzhu (攢竹, BL-2). Cavity located in the depression at the inner ends of the eyebrows.

Zen (忍). To endure. The Japanese name of Chan (禪). See **Chan**.

Zhang, Dao-ling (張道陵). Combined scholarly Daoism with Buddhist philosophies, created religious Daoism (Dao jiao, 道教) sometime during the Chinese Eastern Han dynasty (東漢) (25–221 CE).

zhen zhan (震顫). Press and vibrate.

zheng qi (正氣). Righteous qi.

zhishi (志室, BL-52). Cavity of the lower back.

zhuan fa lun (轉法輪). Turning the wheel of natural law.

Zhuang Zhou (莊周). Contemporary of Mencius. Advocated Daoism.

zhong (忠). Loyalty.

zhongwan (中脘, CV-12). Cavity below the sternum.

zhongfu (中府, LU-1). Cavity on the side of the upper chest.

zu jue yin gan jing (足厥陰肝經). Leg absolute yin liver channel.

zu shao yang dan jing (足少陽膽經). Leg lesser yang gall bladder channel.

zu shao yin shen jing (足少陰腎經). Leg lesser yin kidney channel.

zu tai yang pang guang jing (足太陽膀胱經). Leg greater yang bladder channel.

zu tai yin pi jing (足太陰脾經). Leg greater yin spleen channel.

zu yang ming wei jing (足陽明胃經). Leg yang brightness stomach channel.

zusanli (足三里, ST-36). Cavity of the leg, below the knee.

Index

abdominal deep breathing, 28

Ba Duan Jin, 106, 147, 155
ba mai, 98, 120–121, 147, 150–151
bagua, 96, 147
Baguazhang, 111, 147, 159–160
Bai He, 147, 157–158
baihui, 39–40, 147
baliao, 66–67, 147
binao, 71–73, 147
bu, 68, 111, 147, 149, 153

Chan, 101, 106, 147, 151, 155
changqiang, 66–67, 147
Changquan, 147, 157–158
cheng fo, 109, 147
chengshan, 86–87, 147
chin na, i, 147, 151, 157, 159–161
chize, 82–84, 147
chong mai, 124, 147
Chun Qiu Zhan Guo, 147
circle the waist, 16, 22
circle the tongue to generate saliva, 28
Confucius, 107–108, 148

Da Mo, ii, 110–111, 116, 140, 148, 155, 159
da zhou tian, 101, 105, 148
dan, 17, 93, 99, 102–105, 111, 126–127, 132, 141–143,
     147–150, 152–156
dan ding Dao gong, 143, 148
dan tian, 17, 99, 104–105, 126–127, 141–142, 148, 152,
     154
Dao, 97–98, 108, 142–143, 148–149, 155
Dao De Jing, 108, 148
Dao jia, 108, 148
Dao wai cai yao, 142, 148
Di, 93, 96, 148
di li shi, 96, 148
dian mai, 110, 148
dian qi, 94, 148
dian xue, ix, 29–32, 103, 110, 119, 148, 157
dian xue an mo, 32, 148
Dong Han dynasty, 148
du mai, 105, 120–121, 148

eight vessels, ix, 98, 104, 120–121, 126, 147, 150–151
ermen, 48, 148, 153

feng shui, 96, 148
feng shui shi, 96, 148
fengfu, 51–52, 149
fengshi, 71–73, 149

gongfu, i, 95, 104, 111, 118, 149–151, 153–154, 157–158
gongzhong, 81–82, 149

gui qi, 94, 149
guoshu, 149–150, 153, 157

Han dynasty, 100, 107–108, 139, 148–149, 155
Han, Ching-Tang, 100, 107–108, 139, 148–149, 155, 157
hegu, 68–69, 78–80, 149
Hua Tuo, 106, 149
huantiao, 67, 149
huiyin, 17, 27, 63–64, 149
hukou, 78, 80, 149

jiache, 44–45, 149
jianjing, 52–53, 149
jiankua, 67–68, 149
jianneiling, 54–55, 149
jianyu, 53–54, 149
jiexi, 77–78, 149
jimen, 81–82, 149
Jin, Shao-Feng, 99, 106, 110–111, 140–142, 147–149, 152–153,
     155, 157
jin dan da Dao, 142, 149
jin zhong zhao, 111, 149, 153
jing, 47, 96, 98–99, 101, 105, 108, 110, 120, 127–138,
     140–142, 147–156
jingming, 46, 149
jing qi, 149
jiuwei, 57–59, 149
Jun Qing, 106, 149, 153

kan and li, 112–116
     adjusting, 112, 116
     breathing and
     defined, 93–95, 99, 117
     the mind and, 98, 100, 114–115
     shen and, 116–117, 141–142, 150, 152
     theories of, 93, 112
kong qi, 95, 150
kongzui, 85–86, 150
kufang, 56–57, 150
kuoshu, 150

la ma, 140, 150
Lao Zi, 108, 148, 150
laogong, 90–91, 114, 150
li, vii, 40–41, 53–54, 68–69, 71–76, 78–80, 93, 96, 98,
     112–116, 147–152, 155, 157–158, 160
Li, Shi-Zhen, vii, 40–41, 53–54, 68–69, 71–76, 78–80, 93, 96,
     98, 112–116, 147–152, 155, 157–158, 160
lian jing hua qi, 141, 150
lian shen fan xu, 141, 150
lian qi, 109, 141, 150
lian qi hua shen, 141, 150
Liang dynasty, 110, 150
lieque, 69–70, 88–89, 150
luo, 50, 98, 120, 127, 137, 139, 150, 152

About the Author

Yang, Jwing-Ming, PhD (楊俊敏博士)

Dr. Yang, Jwing-Ming was born on August 11, 1946, in Xinzhu Xian (新竹縣), Taiwan (台灣), Republic of China (中華民國). He started his wushu (武術) (gongfu or kung fu, 功夫) training at the age of fifteen under Shaolin White Crane (Shaolin Bai He, 少林白鶴) Master Cheng, Gin-Gsao (曾金灶). Master Cheng originally learned taizuquan (太祖拳) from his grandfather when he was a child. When Master Cheng was fifteen years old, he started learning White Crane from Master Jin, Shao-Feng (金紹峰) and followed him for twenty-three years until Master Jin's death.

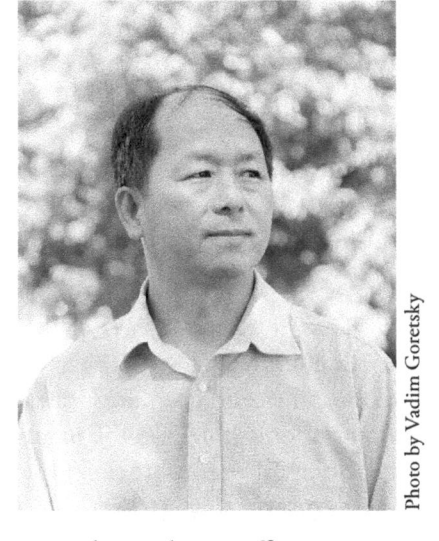

Photo by Vadim Goretsky

In thirteen years of study (1961–1974) under Master Cheng, Dr. Yang became an expert in the White Crane style of Chinese martial arts, which includes both the use of bare hands and various weapons, such as saber, staff, spear, trident, two short rods, and many others. With the same master, he also studied White Crane qigong (氣功), qin na or chin na (擒拿), tui na (推拿), and dian xue massages (點穴按摩) and herbal treatment.

At sixteen, Dr. Yang began the study of Yang-style taijiquan (楊氏太極拳) under Master Kao Tao (高濤). He later continued his study of taijiquan under Master Li, Mao-Ching (李茂清). Master Li learned his taijiquan from the well-known Master Han, Ching-Tang (韓慶堂). From this further practice, Dr. Yang was able to master the taiji bare-hand sequence, pushing hands, the two-man fighting sequence, taiji sword, taiji saber, and taiji qigong.

When Dr. Yang was eighteen years old, he entered Tamkang College (淡江學院) in Taipei Xian to study physics. In college, he began the study of traditional Shaolin Long Fist (Changquan or Chang Chuan, 少林長拳) with Master Li, Mao-Ching at the Tamkang College Guoshu Club (淡江國術社), 1964–1968, and eventually became an assistant instructor under Master Li. In 1971 he completed his MS degree in physics at the National Taiwan University (台灣大學) and then served in the Chinese Air Force from 1971 to 1972. In the service, Dr. Yang taught physics at the Junior Academy of the Chinese Air Force (空軍幼校) while also teaching wushu. After being honorably discharged in 1972, he returned to Tamkang College to teach physics and resumed study under Master Li, Mao-Ching. From Master Li, Dr. Yang learned Northern-style Wushu, which includes bare-hand and kicking techniques as well as numerous weapons.

In 1974 Dr. Yang came to the United States to study mechanical engineering at Purdue University. At the request of a few students, Dr. Yang began to teach gongfu (kung fu), which resulted in the establishment of the Purdue University Chinese Kung Fu Research Club in the spring of 1975. While at Purdue, Dr. Yang also taught college-credit courses in taijiquan. In May 1978, he was awarded a PhD in mechanical engineering by Purdue.

In 1980 Dr. Yang moved to Houston to work for Texas Instruments. While in Houston, he founded Yang's Shaolin Kung Fu Academy, which was eventually taken over by his disciple, Mr. Jeffery Bolt, after Dr. Yang moved to Boston in 1982. Dr. Yang founded Yang's Martial Arts Academy in Boston on October 1, 1982.

In January 1984, he gave up his engineering career to devote more time to research, writing, and teaching. In March 1986, he purchased property in the Jamaica Plain area of Boston to be used as the headquarters of the new organization, Yang's Martial Arts Association (YMAA). The organization expanded to become a division of Yang's Oriental Arts Association, Inc. (YOAA).

In 2008 Dr. Yang began the nonprofit YMAA California Retreat Center. This training facility in rural California is where selected students enroll in a five-year residency to learn Chinese martial arts.

Dr. Yang has been involved in traditional Chinese wushu since 1961, studying Shaolin White Crane (Bai He), Shaolin Long Fist (Changquan), and taijiquan under several different masters. He has taught for more than forty-six years: seven years in Taiwan, five years at Purdue University, two years in Houston, twenty-six years in Boston, and more than eight years at the YMAA California Retreat Center. He has taught seminars all over the world, sharing his knowledge of Chinese martial arts and qigong in Argentina, Austria, Barbados, Botswana, Belgium, Bermuda, Brazil, Canada, China, Chile, England, Egypt, France, Germany, Hungary, Iceland, Ireland, Italy, Latvia, Mexico, the Netherlands, New Zealand, Poland, Portugal, Saudi Arabia, South Africa, Spain, Switzerland, and Venezuela.

Since 1986 YMAA has become an international organization, which currently includes more than fifty schools located in Argentina, Belgium, Canada, Chile, France, Hungary, Iran, Ireland, Italy, New Zealand, Poland, Portugal, South Africa, Sweden, the United Kingdom, the United States, and Venezuela.

Many of Dr. Yang's books and videos have been translated into other languages, such as French, Italian, Spanish, Polish, Czech, Bulgarian, Russian, German, and Hungarian.

Books and Videos by Dr. Yang, Jwing-Ming

Books Alphabetical

Analysis of Shaolin Chin Na, 2nd ed. YMAA Publication Center, 1987, 2004

Ancient Chinese Weapons: A Martial Artist's Guide, 2nd ed. YMAA Publication Center, 1985, 1999

Arthritis Relief: Chinese Qigong for Healing & Prevention, 2nd ed. YMAA Publication Center, 1991, 2005

Back Pain Relief: Chinese Qigong for Healing and Prevention, 2nd ed. YMAA Publication Center, 1997, 2004

Baguazhang: Theory and Applications, 2nd ed. YMAA Publication Center, 1994, 2008

Comprehensive Applications of Shaolin Chin Na: The Practical Defense of Chinese Seizing Arts. YMAA Publication Center, 1995

Essence of Shaolin White Crane. YMAA Publication Center, 1996

How to Defend Yourself. YMAA Publication Center, 1992

Introduction to Ancient Chinese Weapons. Unique Publications, Inc., 1985

Northern Shaolin Sword, 2nd ed. YMAA Publication Center, 1985, 2000

Qigong for Health and Martial Arts, 2nd ed. YMAA Publication Center, 1995, 1998

Qigong Massage: Fundamental Techniques for Health and Relaxation, 2nd ed. YMAA Publication Center, 1992, 2005

Qigong Meditation: Embryonic Breathing. YMAA Publication Center, 2003

Qigong Meditation: Small Circulation. YMAA Publication Center, 2006

Qigong, the Secret of Youth: Da Mo's Muscle/Tendon Changing and Marrow/Brain Washing Qigong, 2nd ed. YMAA Publication Center, 1989, 2000

Root of Chinese Qigong: Secrets of Qigong Training, 2nd ed. YMAA Publication Center, 1989, 2004

Shaolin Chin Na. Unique Publications, Inc., 1980

Shaolin Long Fist Kung Fu. Unique Publications, Inc., 1981

Simple Qigong Exercises for Health: The Eight Pieces of Brocade, 3rd ed. YMAA Publication Center, 1988, 1997, 2013

Tai Chi Ball Qigong: For Health and Martial Arts. YMAA Publication Center, 2010

Tai Chi Chin Na: The Seizing Art of Taijiquan, 2nd ed. YMAA Publication Center, 1995, 2014

Tai Chi Chuan Classical Yang Style: The Complete Long Form and Qigong, 2nd ed. YMAA Publication Center, 1999, 2010

Tai Chi Chuan Martial Applications, 3rd ed. YMAA Publication Center, 1986, 1996, 2015

Tai Chi Chuan Martial Power, 3rd ed. YMAA Publication Center, 1986, 1996, 2015

Tai Chi Qigong: The Internal Foundation of Tai Chi Chuan, 2nd ed. rev. YMAA Publication Center, 1997, 1990, 2013

Tai Chi Secrets of the Ancient Masters: Selected Readings with Commentary. YMAA Publication Center, 1999

Tai Chi Secrets of the Wû and Li Styles: Chinese Classics, Translation, Commentary. YMAA Publication Center, 2001

Tai Chi Secrets of the Wu Style: Chinese Classics, Translation, Commentary. YMAA Publication Center, 2002

Tai Chi Secrets of the Yang Style: Chinese Classics, Translation, Commentary. YMAA Publication Center, 2001

Tai Chi Sword Classical Yang Style: The Complete Long Form, Qigong, and Applications, 2nd ed. YMAA Publication Center, 1999, 2014

Taijiquan Theory of Dr. Yang, Jwing-Ming: The Root of Taijiquan. YMAA Publication Center, 2003

Xingyiquan: Theory and Applications, 2nd ed. YMAA Publication Center, 1990, 2003

Yang Style Tai Chi Chuan. Unique Publications, Inc., 1981

Videos Alphabetical

Advanced Practical Chin Na in Depth. YMAA Publication Center, 2010

Analysis of Shaolin Chin Na. YMAA Publication Center, 2004

Baguazhang (Eight Trigrams Palm Kung Fu). YMAA Publication Center, 2005

Chin Na in Depth: Courses 1–4. YMAA Publication Center, 2003

Chin Na in Depth: Courses 5–8. YMAA Publication Center, 2003

Chin Na in Depth: Courses 9–12. YMAA Publication Center, 2003

Five Animal Sports Qigong. YMAA Publication Center, 2008

Knife Defense: Traditional Techniques. YMAA Publication Center, 2011

Meridian Qigong. YMAA Publication Center, 2015

Neigong. YMAA Publication Center, 2015

Northern Shaolin Sword. YMAA Publication Center, 2009

Qigong Massage. YMAA Publication Center, 2005

Saber Fundamental Training. YMAA Publication Center, 2008

Shaolin Kung Fu Fundamental Training. YMAA Publication Center, 2004

Shaolin Long Fist Kung Fu: Basic Sequences. YMAA Publication Center, 2005

Shaolin Saber Basic Sequences. YMAA Publication Center, 2007

Shaolin Staff Basic Sequences. YMAA Publication Center, 2007

Shaolin White Crane Gong Fu Basic Training: Courses 1 & 2. YMAA Publication Center, 2003

Shaolin White Crane Gong Fu Basic Training: Courses 3 & 4. YMAA Publication Center, 2008

Shaolin White Crane Hard and Soft Qigong. YMAA Publication Center, 2003

Shuai Jiao: Kung Fu Wrestling. YMAA Publication Center, 2010

Simple Qigong Exercises for Arthritis Relief. YMAA Publication Center, 2007

Simple Qigong Exercises for Back Pain Relief. YMAA Publication Center, 2007

Simple Qigong Exercises for Health: The Eight Pieces of Brocade. YMAA Publication Center, 2003

Staff Fundamental Training: Solo Drills and Matching Practice. YMAA Publication Center, 2007

Sword Fundamental Training. YMAA Publication Center, 2009

Tai Chi Ball Qigong: Courses 1 & 2. YMAA Publication Center, 2006

Tai Chi Ball Qigong: Courses 3 & 4. YMAA Publication Center, 2007

Tai Chi Chuan: Classical Yang Style. YMAA Publication Center, 2003

Tai Chi Fighting Set: 2-Person Matching Set. YMAA Publication Center, 2006

Tai Chi Pushing Hands: Courses 1 & 2. YMAA Publication Center, 2005

Tai Chi Pushing Hands: Courses 3 & 4. YMAA Publication Center, 2006

Tai Chi Qigong. YMAA Publication Center, 2005

Tai Chi Sword, Classical Yang Style. YMAA Publication Center, 2005

Tai Chi Symbol: Yin/Yang Sticking Hands. YMAA Publication Center, 2008

Taiji 37 Postures Martial Applications. YMAA Publication Center, 2008

Taiji Chin Na in Depth. YMAA Publication Center, 2009

Taiji Saber: Classical Yang Style. YMAA Publication Center, 2008

Taiji Wrestling: Advanced Takedown Techniques. YMAA Publication Center, 2008

Understanding Qigong, DVD 1: What Is Qigong? The Human Qi Circulatory System. YMAA Publication Center, 2006

Understanding Qigong, DVD 2: Key Points of Qigong & Qigong Breathing. YMAA Publication Center, 2006

Understanding Qigong, DVD 3: Embryonic Breathing. YMAA Publication Center, 2007

Understanding Qigong, DVD 4: Four Seasons Qigong. YMAA Publication Center, 2007

Understanding Qigong, DVD 5: Small Circulation. YMAA Publication Center, 2007

Understanding Qigong, DVD 6: Martial Arts Qigong Breathing. YMAA Publication Center, 2007

Xingyiquan: Twelve Animals Kung Fu and Applications. YMAA Publication Center, 2008

Yang Tai Chi for Beginners. YMAA Publication Center, 2012

YMAA 25-Year Anniversary. YMAA Publication Center, 2009

6 HEALING MOVEMENTS
101 REFLECTIONS ON TAI CHI CHUAN
108 INSIGHTS INTO TAI CHI CHUAN
ADVANCING IN TAE KWON DO
ANALYSIS OF SHAOLIN CHIN NA 2ND ED
ANCIENT CHINESE WEAPONS
THE ART AND SCIENCE OF STAFF FIGHTING
ART OF HOJO UNDO
ARTHRITIS RELIEF, 3D ED.
BACK PAIN RELIEF, 2ND ED.
BAGUAZHANG, 2ND ED.
BRAIN FITNESS
CARDIO KICKBOXING ELITE
CHIN NA IN GROUND FIGHTING
CHINESE FAST WRESTLING
CHINESE FITNESS
CHINESE TUI NA MASSAGE
CHOJUN
COMPREHENSIVE APPLICATIONS OF SHAOLIN CHIN NA
CONFLICT COMMUNICATION
CROCODILE AND THE CRANE: A NOVEL
CUTTING SEASON: A XENON PEARL MARTIAL ARTS THRILLER
DEFENSIVE TACTICS
DESHI: A CONNOR BURKE MARTIAL ARTS THRILLER
DIRTY GROUND
DR. WU'S HEAD MASSAGE
DUKKHA HUNGRY GHOSTS
DUKKHA REVERB
DUKKHA, THE SUFFERING: AN EYE FOR AN EYE
DUKKHA UNLOADED
ENZAN: THE FAR MOUNTAIN, A CONNOR BURKE MARTIAL
    ARTS THRILLER
ESSENCE OF SHAOLIN WHITE CRANE
EXPLORING TAI CHI
FACING VIOLENCE
FIGHT BACK
FIGHT LIKE A PHYSICIST
THE FIGHTER'S BODY
FIGHTER'S FACT BOOK
FIGHTER'S FACT BOOK 2
FIGHTING THE PAIN RESISTANT ATTACKER
FIRST DEFENSE
FORCE DECISIONS: A CITIZENS GUIDE
FOX BORROWS THE TIGER'S AWE
INSIDE TAI CHI
KAGE: THE SHADOW, A CONNOR BURKE MARTIAL ARTS
    THRILLER
KATA AND THE TRANSMISSION OF KNOWLEDGE
KRAV MAGA PROFESSIONAL TACTICS
KRAV MAGA WEAPON DEFENSES
LITTLE BLACK BOOK OF VIOLENCE
LIUHEBAFA FIVE CHARACTER SECRETS
MARTIAL ARTS ATHLETE
MARTIAL ARTS INSTRUCTION
MARTIAL WAY AND ITS VIRTUES
MASK OF THE KING
MEDITATIONS ON VIOLENCE
MERIDIAN QIGONG EXERCISES
MIND/BODY FITNESS
THE MIND INSIDE TAI CHI
THE MIND INSIDE YANG STYLE TAI CHI CHUAN
MUGAI RYU
NATURAL HEALING WITH QIGONG
NORTHERN SHAOLIN SWORD, 2ND ED.
OKINAWA'S COMPLETE KARATE SYSTEM: ISSHIN RYU
POWER BODY
PRINCIPLES OF TRADITIONAL CHINESE MEDICINE
QIGONG FOR HEALTH & MARTIAL ARTS 2ND ED.

QIGONG FOR LIVING
QIGONG FOR TREATING COMMON AILMENTS
QIGONG MASSAGE
QIGONG MEDITATION: EMBRYONIC BREATHING
QIGONG MEDITATION: SMALL CIRCULATION
QIGONG, THE SECRET OF YOUTH: DA MO'S CLASSICS
QUIET TEACHER: A XENON PEARL MARTIAL ARTS THRILLER
RAVEN'S WARRIOR
REDEMPTION
ROOT OF CHINESE QIGONG, 2ND ED.
SCALING FORCE
SENSEI: A CONNOR BURKE MARTIAL ARTS THRILLER
SHIHAN TE: THE BUNKAI OF KATA
SHIN GI TAI: KARATE TRAINING FOR BODY, MIND, AND SPIRIT
SIMPLE CHINESE MEDICINE
SIMPLE QIGONG EXERCISES FOR HEALTH, 3RD ED.
SIMPLIFIED TAI CHI CHUAN, 2ND ED.
SIMPLIFIED TAI CHI FOR BEGINNERS
SOLO TRAINING
SOLO TRAINING 2
SUDDEN DAWN: THE EPIC JOURNEY OF BODHIDHARMA
SUMO FOR MIXED MARTIAL ARTS
SUNRISE TAI CHI
SUNSET TAI CHI
SURVIVING ARMED ASSAULTS
TAE KWON DO: THE KOREAN MARTIAL ART
TAEKWONDO BLACK BELT POOMSAE
TAEKWONDO: A PATH TO EXCELLENCE
TAEKWONDO: ANCIENT WISDOM FOR THE MODERN
    WARRIOR
TAEKWONDO: DEFENSES AGAINST WEAPONS
TAEKWONDO: SPIRIT AND PRACTICE
TAO OF BIOENERGETICS
TAI CHI BALL QIGONG: FOR HEALTH AND MARTIAL ARTS
TAI CHI BALL WORKOUT FOR BEGINNERS
TAI CHI BOOK
TAI CHI CHIN NA: THE SEIZING ART OF TAI CHI CHUAN, 2ND
    ED.
TAI CHI CHUAN CLASSICAL YANG STYLE, 2ND ED.
TAI CHI CHUAN MARTIAL APPLICATIONS
TAI CHI CHUAN MARTIAL POWER, 3RD ED.
TAI CHI CONNECTIONS
TAI CHI DYNAMICS
TAI CHI FOR DEPRESSION
TAI CHI IN 10 WEEKS
TAI CHI QIGONG, 3RD ED.
TAI CHI SECRETS OF THE ANCIENT MASTERS
TAI CHI SECRETS OF THE WU & LI STYLES
TAI CHI SECRETS OF THE WU STYLE
TAI CHI SECRETS OF THE YANG STYLE
TAI CHI SWORD: CLASSICAL YANG STYLE, 2ND ED.
TAI CHI SWORD FOR BEGINNERS
TAI CHI WALKING
TAIJIQUAN THEORY OF DR. YANG, JWING-MING
TENGU: THE MOUNTAIN GOBLIN, A CONNOR BURKE
    MARTIAL ARTS THRILLER
TIMING IN THE FIGHTING ARTS
TRADITIONAL CHINESE HEALTH SECRETS
TRADITIONAL TAEKWONDO
TRAINING FOR SUDDEN VIOLENCE
WAY OF KATA
WAY OF KENDO AND KENJITSU
WAY OF SANCHIN KATA
WAY TO BLACK BELT
WESTERN HERBS FOR MARTIAL ARTISTS
WILD GOOSE QIGONG
WOMAN'S QIGONG GUIDE
XINGYIQUAN

DVDS FROM YMAA

ADVANCED PRACTICAL CHIN NA IN-DEPTH
ANALYSIS OF SHAOLIN CHIN NA
ATTACK THE ATTACK
BAGUAZHANG: EMEI BAGUAZHANG
BEGINNER QIGONG FOR WOMEN
CHEN STYLE TAIJIQUAN
CHIN NA IN-DEPTH COURSES 1—4
CHIN NA IN-DEPTH COURSES 5—8
CHIN NA IN-DEPTH COURSES 9—12
FACING VIOLENCE: 7 THINGS A MARTIAL ARTIST MUST KNOW
FIVE ANIMAL SPORTS
JOINT LOCKS
KNIFE DEFENSE: TRADITIONAL TECHNIQUES AGAINST A DAGGER
KUNG FU BODY CONDITIONING 1
KUNG FU BODY CONDITIONING 2
KUNG FU FOR KIDS
KUNG FU FOR TEENS
INFIGHTING
LOGIC OF VIOLENCE
MERIDIAN QIGONG
NEIGONG FOR MARTIAL ARTS
NORTHERN SHAOLIN SWORD : SAN CAI JIAN, KUN WU JIAN, QI MEN JIAN
QIGONG MASSAGE
QIGONG FOR CANCER
QIGONG FOR HEALING
QIGONG FOR LONGEVITY
QIGONG FOR WOMEN
SABER FUNDAMENTAL TRAINING
SAI TRAINING AND SEQUENCES
SANCHIN KATA: TRADITIONAL TRAINING FOR KARATE POWER
SHAOLIN KUNG FU FUNDAMENTAL TRAINING: COURSES 1 & 2
SHAOLIN LONG FIST KUNG FU: BASIC SEQUENCES
SHAOLIN LONG FIST KUNG FU: INTERMEDIATE SEQUENCES
SHAOLIN LONG FIST KUNG FU: ADVANCED SEQUENCES 1
SHAOLIN LONG FIST KUNG FU: ADVANCED SEQUENCES 2
SHAOLIN SABER: BASIC SEQUENCES
SHAOLIN STAFF: BASIC SEQUENCES
SHAOLIN WHITE CRANE GONG FU BASIC TRAINING: COURSES 1 & 2
SHAOLIN WHITE CRANE GONG FU BASIC TRAINING: COURSES 3 & 4
SHUAI JIAO: KUNG FU WRESTLING
SIMPLE QIGONG EXERCISES FOR ARTHRITIS RELIEF
SIMPLE QIGONG EXERCISES FOR BACK PAIN RELIEF
SIMPLIFIED TAI CHI CHUAN: 24 & 48 POSTURES

SIMPLIFIED TAI CHI FOR BEGINNERS 48
SUNRISE TAI CHI
SUNSET TAI CHI
SWORD: FUNDAMENTAL TRAINING
TAEKWONDO KORYO POOMSAE
TAI CHI BALL QIGONG: COURSES 1 & 2
TAI CHI BALL QIGONG: COURSES 3 & 4
TAI CHI BALL WORKOUT FOR BEGINNERS
TAI CHI CHUAN CLASSICAL YANG STYLE
TAI CHI CONNECTIONS
TAI CHI ENERGY PATTERNS
TAI CHI FIGHTING SET
TAI CHI FIT FLOW
TAI CHI FIT OVER 50
TAI CHI FIT STRENGTH
TAI CHI FIT TO GO
TAI CHI FOR WOMEN
TAI CHI PUSHING HANDS: COURSES 1 & 2
TAI CHI PUSHING HANDS: COURSES 3 & 4
TAI CHI SWORD: CLASSICAL YANG STYLE
TAI CHI SWORD FOR BEGINNERS
TAI CHI SYMBOL: YIN YANG STICKING HANDS
TAIJI & SHAOLIN STAFF: FUNDAMENTAL TRAINING
TAIJI CHIN NA IN-DEPTH
TAIJI 37 POSTURES MARTIAL APPLICATIONS
TAIJI SABER CLASSICAL YANG STYLE
TAIJI WRESTLING
TRAINING FOR SUDDEN VIOLENCE
UNDERSTANDING QIGONG 1: WHAT IS QI? • HUMAN QI CIRCULATORY SYSTEM
UNDERSTANDING QIGONG 2: KEY POINTS • QIGONG BREATHING
UNDERSTANDING QIGONG 3: EMBRYONIC BREATHING
UNDERSTANDING QIGONG 4: FOUR SEASONS QIGONG
UNDERSTANDING QIGONG 5: SMALL CIRCULATION
UNDERSTANDING QIGONG 6: MARTIAL QIGONG BREATHING
WHITE CRANE HARD & SOFT QIGONG
WUDANG KUNG FU: FUNDAMENTAL TRAINING
WUDANG SWORD
WUDANG TAIJIQUAN
XINGYIQUAN
YANG TAI CHI FOR BEGINNERS
YMAA 25 YEAR ANNIVERSARY DVD

more products available from . . .
YMAA Publication Center, Inc. 楊氏東方文化出版中心
1-800-669-8892 • info@ymaa.com • www.ymaa.com

Printed in the USA
CPSIA information can be obtained
at www.ICGtesting.com
JSHW060041150824
68134JS00028B/2582

9 781594 3941